NELL'S
JOURNEY

Wyatt House books may be ordered through booksellers or by contacting:

WYATT HOUSE PUBLISHING
399 Lakeview Dr. W.
Mobile, Alabama 36695
www.wyattpublishing.com
editor@wyattpublishing.com

Because of the dynamic nature of the Internet, any web address or links contained in this book may have changed since publication and may no longer be valid.

Cover and interior design by: Mark Wyatt

ISBN 13: 978-1-7326049-2-6

Printed in the United States of America

NELL'S JOURNEY

A CAREGIVER'S MEMOIR OF ALZHEIMER'S

DR. BILL WHITFIELD

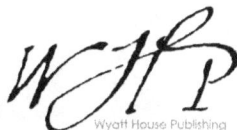

Wyatt House Publishing

Mobile, Alabama

Nell was discovered to have Alzheimer's in the summer of 2014, and it has progressed to such a point that I have decided to keep a journal. One thing that has been beneficial at the beginning was to meet as a family with a retired Alzheimer's counselor, to discuss the legal aspects of Nell's Alzheimer's disease and what to do while Nell was still lucid enough to understand what legal papers she needed to sign now, so when the time came and she was not able to comprehend, the legal things were already completed. This counselor was the Gulf Coast representative for the Alzheimer's Association for a number of years and was the greatest help to us, and looking back, she is appreciated, for her counsel.

As I was editing this diary, I realized that I included a lot of personal things about my caregiving experiences as the Alzheimer's began to take its daily toll in Nell's life. I was tempted to edit a lot of that out of my diary. Then as I thought about it, I decided to leave these experiences in because I wanted to be real in my diary. I wanted to share the daily hardships and trying times. I wanted to share the decisions I made not to put

Nell in a nursing home, then thinking I should. Often, I felt I would try to justify my thoughts about putting her into a nursing home because it was best for Nell. Then I would realize, that I wanted to put her into a nursing home because it would be best for me. I tried to share some of my feelings, emotional experiences and spiritual trying times. Looking back, I think I could have done a much better job of caregiving than what I did. I wanted to put this diary into print for an Alzheimer's caregiver to read in order to give the person what could be ahead in their caregiving responsibilities.

On October 26, 2017 I was cleaning my desktop computer and came across some notes I made of Nell's peculiar actions (Personality changes) way before we had any idea of her having Alzheimer's disease. I have inserted some of these notes below. I titled them: "A Loving Account" at the time. I was somewhat upset with her at various occasions by her actions, not knowing what was going on in her personality "change." Some of the notes I wrote at the time was not included in this diary.

It all came on me in this near auto accident that something was not just right with Nell's usually sharp mental processes. She was driving us on I-65 to Dauphin Way Baptist Church between Springhill and Dauphin St., going south when the cars ahead slowed to a near stop, and Nell did not appear to be aware of this traffic problem ahead. I looked at her and she was looking straight ahead at the stoppage, yet she did not attempt to stop but, appeared to me, to be in a daze. I shouted for her to put the brakes on, which she did immediately.

I discussed this with family. It was agreed for her to see a neurologist. She consented, because she seemed to be aware that something was going on with her mental processes. Nell saw a neurologist, on Sept. 25th 2013. He had her do a number of tests, which included blood, and an MRI. In a follow up visit he told us that she did not have any of the normal patterns

Bill Whitfield

that indicated signs of Alzheimer's. She feared that and was relieved with that diagnosis. The doctor said he could detect in the tests that there were signs of aging. This did not satisfy me. She was 77 and should show signs of aging. I didn't think this would describe her personality changes.

After the near accident, I began to recall a number of different things that had been happening. I remembered the time some months before, she was driving to WalMart in Tillman's Corner when she turned in front of a pickup truck going into Walmart and it hit her so hard, that she fell over the rider's side and her foot hit the accelerator and she drove across the street in a plowed ground and settled there. Her mobile telephone was on the right side floor board and it dialed my phone. I was just getting ready to do a graveside funeral at Pinecrest Cemetery when I received her call. She did not call. The phone called by "accident" and I could hear the EMS responders talking to her. I heard her responding, but neither the responders nor Nell knew that I could hear what was going on. They told her they were taking her to the Knollwood Hospital Emergency. I could not leave the cemetery at that moment, so I called my daughter to go to the Knollwood emergency to meet Nell at the hospital. Nell banged her head pretty hard and later I thought, that could have been the start of her dementia. Soon after that, we were driving out the driveway at our house in Cypress Shores on our bicycles and she drove her bicycle straight into some Azalea bushes and bruised and cut herself. When I thought back to those things, I realized that she could have been in a physical state of dementia at that time.

There were many other signs after looking back, that could have given me a clue. After some examination later by the doctor I thought at the time there were responses that were not ordinary, both in word or deed on occasion. Since the visit to the doctor I had given more attention to the odd things she says or does. Nell will be completely normal, and then, as if she slips a mental cog, she will say or do something that is not her

7

usual bright self. For instance, we will be in agreement to go to a certain place, and in a few minutes she will be talking about going to this other place with no remembrance of our previous conversation and agreement. I didn't make an issue of it and went right on. This has happened in various ways, with different events and places. It is not a big problem, just perplexing. I do believe that she was aware of it, and was concerned, and caused her worry, and she kept it in her heart. I entered the bedroom after we came in from Ruth Chris Restaurant, having our 59th wedding anniversary dinner. She was nearly undressed for bed, and sitting on the sofa chair with her head in her hands. It was more than praying. It was an emotional hurt for me to see her. I don't remember if I said anything to her about it, at the time.

When we parked outside of Ruth Chris' Restaurant prior to going in, we agreed what we were going to order to come under the amount of the gift certificate the church had given us in recognition of our 15 year tenure at Dauphin Way. Our decisions were, she was going to get a petite filet, and I was going to order a T-bone steak. Before the waiter came as we were looking at the menu she decided on a T-bone steak, also. When I was giving the order to the waiter, of two T-bone steaks, she said, "No, I want a petite filet.!" When the waiter asked how she wanted it cooked, it went like this: "I want it well done." I said: "Are you sure you don't want a little pink?" She said to the waiter, "Yes, with a little pink. You know what I mean", just throwing the decision off as a "matter of fact" attitude. There was more involved, as I think, the waiter felt he was dealing with someone with some senility. That was my impression, of course.

Nell has tried to compensate during the day in our relationship by a different personality. She is trying to be upbeat and full of life and excitement. Even when she is around the office staff personnel she says things, to me I know, that are a little off her normal responses, like she has to say something, no matter what comes from her lips.

In most cases the problems in her thinking and talking is noticed by me, as far as I know, not by others. No one has said anything, they all seemed to like her, and I think they just say: "That Nell is something isn't she?" She is normal in her life, during the day, except at times something unusual happens that I realize is not normal, but the rest of the day, all is well.

THE BEGINNING

10/31/13   We just returned on 10/29 from a trip to California to see my family. Nell and I attended my 65 class Reunion. An event with Nell's thought process left me bewildered. I did not answer a call on my cell phone from Kentucky. "Later" I said "I might answer it". The phone number came up on the screen. Nell said there would be no use to call it because it would go to a dead end. It would go into a wasteland. I asked her what sense that made. I asked if she ever called that number before. She said no. She begin having trouble with her phone. My son Billy bought her a phone on his account that was easier for her to use. She had trouble with it also. (I finally I had to cancel it).

11/6/13   When we left a church member's funeral to go to the their residence for a fellowship meal with the family and friends I asked Nell to find the address on the GPS. She had put addresses in the GPS many times before. This time however she was confused, and couldn't put it in. I finally did it myself.

After I had led the widow and widower's class later in that same day we were going home to pack up for the Gulf, and driving across I-65 on Dauphin St she asked me if I saw that flash ahead in the sky. I was looking where she was looking and did not see it. I said (to myself) it must have been in her eyes. I meant a mind thing. "Maybe you need to get your eyes checked?" I think she knew what I meant. She wanted me to know it was something which was of concern to her, otherwise she would not have mentioned it. I think it may have happened before, and because she was concerned, she wanted me to know. She blurted out, "I am not going to the doctor!", meaning the neurologist.

I need patience because 99 % of the time she is normal and then in a moment she says or does something that is out of the ordinary for her. She has become more sweet and submissive in her personality. At times she is more talkative and lively, but I have to be aware and need to correct what she says. If it doesn't make any difference I just let it go.

2016

3/22/16   In my devotion today, in the book _124 Prayers for Caregivers_, by Joan Guntzelman, the subjects daily are in caregiving, and helping the patient to continue on their journey in life. How blessed one can be in being a part of another person's journey. I am the caregiver for Nell in her journey in life. Now she has Alzheimer's, and requires constant care for all her needs in our journey. Last night I was helping Nell get out of the bathtub at our son Billy's Gulf Shores home at the Martinique. The tub was deeper than the tub we have at our house in Saraland, and it was quite difficult to get her on her feet in the tub. I tried to get her to stand in the tub, then I could help her step over the edge safely. She was just about on her feet, and then slipped back down into the tub of water. She said, "Oh, oh!" I took her to mean, that her trusting in me to get her out of the tub has failed, and now she is in trouble. I finally was able to work with her to get her out, and get her in bed. In the morning as I reflected on that bath experience, and thinking about her journey, I was recalling the times in our 62 years, she trusted me to take care of her on her journey. Now, however, if I couldn't get her out, she would have to stay there. She trusted in me to get her out. She could not think beyond that. Of course, I could always call on help. She was only

13

thinking of me, if I would be able to get her out of the tub. Nell has had quite a journey in life. She came from a home where she was loved by all her aunts and uncles, and cousins. She was from a home where the finances were very limited. Her mother and aunts sewed most of her clothes. She was born in Mobile, Al., and was taken to church in the nursery at Dauphin Way Baptist Church, at Ann and Dauphin St.in Mobile, Al, right after she was born. The parents, in those days, never seemed to have any problem with taking their new born to church as soon as the mother was able to attend church. She was reared in the church. They attended Sunday morning, Sunday night and Wednesday night.

SPEAKING A WHOLE THOUGHT BECOMES DIFFICULT

We were eating breakfast on the patio one morning. Nell was not able to speak a complete thought at this time. She would mostly "parrot" things others would say. If we walked by a table at a restaurant, and she overheard a person at a table while we passed by, say something, Nell would repeat it out loud and the person who said the thing that Nell repeated would look at her in a kind of insulting manner, thinking that Nell was mocking her. But Nell did it in such a nonchalant way in walking right by, that the person would quickly realize that things were not "right" with Nell, and usually, they would smile.

Continuing my comment, while we were eating, just out of the blue, Nell looked at me and said "You look just like Jesus." I was so shocked that she had a complete thought, and that in that complete thought, she said such a thing, that I was overwhelmed at her statement. I thought to myself: I have tried not to do anything that would hurt her feelings, even if she went to the potty at an inconvenient place and time, or forgetting to replace her Depends when she went to the potty, and wet the kitchen chair or her sofa chair because she did not put her depends on. I would just go and clean up the wet and put the chair in the sun to dry. She would be nonchalant about it, and sit and watch TV, or go sit on the patio, oblivious to what she did, or no worry that I was cleaning up her "problem."

If I smelled that she had an "accident", I would say: "Did you go to the potty in your Depends? She would say: "Potty." Then, I would remove her clothes, take her into the shower and clean her, and put Depends and clean clothes on her, and she would not have any misgivings, apology, or express any remorse, but would be an obedient "object," that was being cleaned. When cleaned we would continue what we were doing. There was nothing emotional about it. It was just something that was done in the usual activities of the day.

5/29/2016   When I got up this morning, I had a difficult time sleeping during the night. I was overwhelmed with a dark, negative feeling. I was trying to think what I needed to do first in the morning. First, I was to get breakfast ready. Shall I get Nell showered and dressed first, or feed her first? I began showering Nell in the morning, because she would wear her Depends all night and she would not smell pleasant. So, I would normally shower her first and dress her, and then have breakfast. When I was doing my devotion and praying, I felt so lonely. I just needed friends or family, or acquaintances or someone to talk to, to be around. It is a miracle that after my devotion and prayer, I had an overwhelming joy come over my heart that I had a "presence" and the opportunity to minister to Nell another day to make life pleasant for her - on her journey. It was also my journey.

Many times in the night I would have negative feelings, an indescribable sense of disgust with life, of hopelessness, of darkness, not only emotional, but physical with stomach sickness. Even while sleeping – there is a disgust in my gut (the only words I know to describe my feeling) behind my unconsciousness. I am not resting but tossing and turning. Then being brought to full consciousness find that several hours, maybe four or five, have passed. I thought I was awake, in my tossing, but I was actually asleep. I usually get up about 5:00 A.M., and I am glad to look at the clock and see it is 5:00 A.M. If it is 4:00 A.M. I am disappointed, and try to sleep till 5:00, but finally get up at 4:30 A.M. As far as I can tell, there is no negative feelings directed toward Nell; nor directed toward God. It is just a feeling I am experiencing within myself. I am a cacoon, and outside of my person, I seem to be related alright, but within myself, I have a sickness, mentally and physically. After some time and activity, I come out and feel good, mentally and physically.

5/30/2016   I am overwhelmed this morning with the thought that my whole life -- outside a few short years have been with my companion Nell. Every thought – action or re-action to everything , included her. Every event she was in my mind with the event. Many times she was the central figure – child bearing in all its aspects. Bearing children in all of its ramifications and tending to the necessities from morning to night – every day – from morning to night, year after year. When I went to work she sent me on my way, cared for me as I departed into my world, both as pilot, as salesman, as student, as minister, she was by my side, in full support and encour-agement. She did not say, "Poor me, you are gone all day, and I have had to take care of the children. She would not say: "Now you get in here and give them their supper and give them their bath." I would do that from time to time, but there was not any nagging or complaint about her daily task of child rear-ing. In decisions we were together, even though, ultimately, I made them, - she was dominant, (she was in the equation-in an important manner) but subservient and encouraging. Now, here we are, still together – she dominates , yet is subservient and cooperative in her illness as I care for her needs with all my heart and no regrets, for we are one. This is the "Today the

Lord has made, I will rejoice and be glad in it." This is the life the Lord has given to us. Life, to some, go in other ways, but this is the stage of life we have – we are only to respond as best we can, with God's help.

5/31/2016 While sleeping, I can feel a negative, dark, hurtful feeling come over my body and mind. I have noticed that when Nell rolls over in bed and puts her leg over me as she used to do prior to her sickness, I have a different feeling come over me. One of well-being, like she is alright now—she is getting better. Then when I get her up, she is still the same. I cope with it, and try to make her day start out with a cheerful greeting.

6/2/2016 Last night as I got Nell to bed, there were several problems, that occurred while she got ready for bed. I have to be quite attentive, because about a month ago, as she was drying herself, and I was hanging her clothes in the closet, she fell backwards in the tub and hit her head, and blood just gushed out. I got her out of the tub, and cleaned her up. She seemed alright after awhile, so I didn't take her to the hospital. Several days later, I put her in the bath tub and she layed back resting her head on the tub. When I came to get her out of the bath, she was semi-conscious. I got her out of the tub, but had to call my daughter to come help me get her on her feet to get her into bed. She became quite conscious after about 15 minutes, so I did not take her to the hospital.

So, last night I tried to be more attentive and may have tried to be more restrictive in her moving around before I helped her in bed. I am sure she realized that she was giving me some extra trouble, and finally I got her in bed and she layed her head on her pillow. I leaned over her, and said, "I love you," and kissed her on the forehead. She said, " I am just a sinner, saved by grace." I just about fainted to hear her say a long sentence and a complete thought. I said, "I am too." There are daily events that are surprising, difficult, humorous, but it is just life with a loved one with the illness Alzheimers.

6/4/2016 (Sat) Friday, I took Nell to E.A. Roberts, (a day care facility for Alzheimer's patients) about 8:15 A.M. I played golf with several men from Dauphin Way Baptist Church. We completed our game about 1:30 P.M. I went home, warmed up a piece of pizza left over from several days prior. I showered and took a nap. I went to pick up Nell at 5 :00 P.M. from E.A. Roberts. I noticed "right off", that Nell had a somber demeanor. She wore a visor cap, she decorated during the day. Driving to dinner, her attitude was somber. We visited Carrie after we ate. Her attitude was somber. After about 45 minutes, I asked if she was ready to go home. She jumped up and headed to the door to leave. It was about 8:15 PM., which was the time I normally get Nell ready for bed. We got home, she went into the bedroom from the bathroom after she took her pills, and brushed her teeth. I helped her get into her night gown. All this time, she was different from her normal demeanor, one of somber face and attitude. She had no smile. I leaned over her and said: "I love you." She responded, rather curtly, "I love you." In attempting to describe our relationship, from the time I picked her up from E.A. Roberts to her laying in bed to sleep, was one of separateness. I am fearful of a relationship of unrecognizing me, not the normal warmth in our relationship. I don't know if she resented me being gone for so long as she was at E. A. Roberts. She seems to like going there.

This is day 18 of taking Namenda, on the advice of Nell's neurologist. I am worried that it is not helping, and when Nell stops taking the medicine after 28 days of the sample kit, she may be far worse than when she began. As her husband and caregiver , I ask myself if I am doing wrong to consent to have Nell take these Alzheimer pills? An Alzheimer counselor, whom I respect, recommends not taking any of the Alzheimer medicine. But, I feel like I am betraying Nell by not doing all I can to help her in her life. Nell's neurologist assures me that they help, but I can't see it. Maybe she would be worse off if I didn't give her the pills.

6/7/2016   Sometimes, "just out of the blue," Nell completes a whole sentence of a thought she has on her mind. Other times, she starts out to tell me something and her mind just shuts down after a few words. Some days she seems alert to her environment, and other times she just wants to sit or lay on the couch and sleep. There are times, she says or does things, that prompts me to think the doctors have misdiagnosed her dementia; that it is not Alzheimers, but something that can be healed. Maybe, I think, it is a urinary track infection, and can be treated and she can be normal again. Nell is so kind, so patient in responding to my care. I thank God for that, it seems as if she knows she has a "problem," and tries to cooperate in every way to make it "easy" on me. When she "messes" her Depends and clothes, on the floor and toilet, she just stands to make it easy for me to clean her and put clean clothes on her, and clean up the bathroom. When I put her in the shower, she turns as I give her instruction so l can reach all parts of her body to soap and rinse her from outside the shower area.

6/8/2016   Nell and I went to the senior center in Saraland for lunch Wednesday. We try to eat lunch at the senior center several times a week. Every body has their place at the various tables. When we come, we sit across from several widow Christian ladies about 70 years of age. That is our place. They want us to sit with them. One of the ladies made a comment that they thought I was a good husband the way I took care of Nell. They commended me. I am only doing what I ought to be doing and was astonished that they commended me. Not only doing what I ought to be doing, but would not feel good, not doing for Nell in taking care of her needs.

6/10/2016   This morning Nell spent some time in the toilet area before breakfast, then we ate an omelet I made. I gave her a shower and got her dressed for the day. We were getting ready to go to Big Level, Ms., and I told Nell to go to the bathroom before we left. After she went into the bathroom for a while, I went in to check if all was alright. She had "messed" up her Depends, her pants, her lower body. I had to get her into the shower and get new Depends and pants on before we could leave.

6/12/2016   This is Sunday morning. Last night I was typing on my laptop at the dining room table. Nell was watching TV, "OJ vs Public" in her chair. I could see her. Carrie came by and I went to the door to let her in and noticed Nell was not in her chair. I went to look for her in the bedroom. She had gone to the bathroom area and took off all her clothes and got in bed. I then, got her into her pajamas, put on her Depends and gave her, her night time medicine and put her back in bed.

That was Saturday night, Sunday morning I found myself yearning for the time when Nell was so full of life. I can hardly remember her that way after ministering to her with her Alzheimers for two years. Now she is entirely different. I am down mentally, thinking that the way she is now is how I remember her and know her. I feel bad about that. 62 years of marriage and I know her as she is now in these last two years. Day by day she becomes more of a shell of a person. From time to time there are moments of her "old" self.

Last night when I got into bed she turned over towards me and stuttered – very stumbling, hardly completing her thought and finally got it out. She said, "I love you very much." Just to reflect on that complete thought this morning, brings tears to my eyes. Soon, I will be in another day of caregiving when she gets up, and not knowing what I will deal with. But I will be patient, and loving, with God's help.

EATING BECOMES DIFFICULT

PM of the same day: We went to lunch today at Olive Gardens. A mixed marriage couple with a child sat next to us. Nell just stared at them. It was difficult for her to eat. I like to eat out, because I can't cook, nor plan meals well. But it is very difficult to eat out with Nell's difficulty and slow to eat. So, I don't know what to do. She will use the fingers on her left hand to help put food on her fork, and sometimes it spills on her dress. It makes a big mess on her dress, so we can't go anywhere else afterwards. When I can I put a towel or something else to make a bib to keep her dress clean.

6/21/2016   See, but do not perceive, I read in the devotion today. One thing—I do not see God in things around me, in people, events, actions, and circumstances as He is, and as I used to, at times so clearly. Satan seems to attack in so many ways when you are an attentive caregiver. I feel sometimes, the relief I yearn for, would come, if God would be gracious and take me to Himself. At times, doubts come in my mind about God, Jesus, the Bible.

People say they care and If I need any help to ask them. They would help, I know, but I am afraid to ask, because they may refuse for some good reason, that they can't help that day or hour.

I hurt my arm, and it hindered my caregiving ability. I wondered, what would happen to Nell and I, if I was completely disabled, physically, or worse, mentally? The children are kind, concerned, but they have their lives and children and grandchildren to tend to and help. We are elderly and loved, but –maybe—a bother—at times.

6/22/2016   Nell and I went to lunch at Pintoli's Restaurant in Satsuma, yesterday with Dauphin Way members from Chickasaw. Nell had a hard time eating. She dropped food from her fork on her dress. I need to feed her when we go out, because she takes so long to get food on a fork and raise it to her mouth. She uses fingers on her left hand to help get the food on her fork.

It is interesting how her mind works. While we were eating, a mutual acquaintance was mentioned, but we could only remember the first names of the husband and wife. Nell just came up with the last name, right out of the "blue." It was amazing. She was listening to the conversation and just jumped right in with the name. It shows she was aware of what was being said. You don't think she is aware. I ask her later on occasions: "Did you enjoy yourself today?" She will say: "I enjoyed myself."

Last night she had a hard time getting into bed. She got half way up and just stopped. She wouldn't move when I tried to assist. Finally, she pushed herself up and layed her head on the pillow. She can't get up without my help, at least not safely. She is too unsteady. I am afraid she will fall and hit her head on the night stand, or injure herself another way.

My own feelings today as we begin a new day, worries me that she may reveal a worse condition mentally and physically different than yesterday. It is emotionally, very hurtful to see these differences, when they are revealed. Several days ago, twice, she would go and sit in the car, as if we were going somewhere.

After supper last night, about 7:15 PM, we were watching the news on television. She just got up from her chair and began walking to the bedroom. I asked her: "Where are you going?" She answered: "Where are you going?" I asked her: "Are you tired?" She answered: "Tired." I said, "Do you want to go to bed?" She answered: "Go to sleepy."

I can't express my feelings as I get her ready for bed. She is kind and patient. She just passively stands as I put her gown on her. I see that she takes her medicine and brushes her teeth. I say to her while she lies in bed, "I love you." She responds with such true thankfulness, with emotion in her words, "I Love you," with the full meaning of the words to express her love. It is tough to see; your wife, your lover, mother to our children, partner in ministry, helpmeet in life, fade away from life, little by little, day by day. God is my strength, He meets me in so many occasions to give me strength to care for her in a loving manner. I pray to stay healthy so to give her the best of care, before He takes me, or I am physically or mentally unable to do it. Certainly I would want to give her the best of care before she doesn't know who I am, and, of course, if she goes to be with the Lord before me.

6/25/16   We have Nell's cousin and wife with us for a few days. She grew up with him. He was always a cousin who Nell had warm memories of after she grew up. She hasn't seen him much through the years but she knew him and his brother. We all met at Olive Gardens last night and had a good visit and meal. We got to bed later than usual last night. Today, she has not been as aware as she usually is. She seems to be "down" or maybe depressed. She has tried to say things, to complete a thought several times, but then she stops and blows air out of her pursed lips. Her mind goes to another world. She just stares forward. I know it is frustrating, but her mind deals with it someway. She has wanted to sleep more today. It is 4:00 PM on Saturday, and she has been sleeping for about an hour. She slept about an hour after we returned from shopping about 12:30. After we had lunch she went back to the bed to take a nap.

6/7/2016 Tuesday, when I picked up Nell at E. A. Roberts, Nell had a blood pressure of 165/108. The nurse told me to take it at night and again in the morning, which I did. It was 165/61, and about the same, when I took it again in the morning. I talked to our doctor's nurse, and she said the doctor advised to continue taking her blood pressure and it may be that he might have to change her blood pressure medicine.

We have been going for a walk in the afternoon to the end of our street and back again. She is tired and sits in her chair while watching TV, after we return. She has been feeling good today, although while at Rocky Creek Catfish Restaurant, I had to mostly feed her. She is getting where it is becoming more difficult for her to get the food to her mouth. It becomes so difficult at times, that she picks up food with her fingers. She will get food on her utinsel, and just holds it, without putting it into her mouth. It is easier for me to feed her than watch her try to feed herself. It is nerve wracking and painful to watch her.

7/10/16 We had a full day of activities Saturday. We went to the funeral of a member of Dauphin Way Baptist Church. I was part of the Men's Prayer group's honorary pallbearers. A friend sat with Nell and took her to the bathroom before we left the church area. We met friends for lunch. This was difficult because Nell is not able to eat well. She cannot lift the fork to her mouth. It usually results in my feeding her.

We went to visit Bill's place in Big Level, Ms. His family was there. Stacey & Trey with Emma. Will and Mick were there from Mississippi State. Anita was busy unpacking. We visited for several hours and left. We ate supper at Rocky Creek Catfish Restaurant in Lucedale. I had to, mostly, feed Nell. We arrived home in Saraland about 8:30 P.M. Nell went to bed when we got home.

This Sunday morning I got Nell up about 7:00 A. M. She had an accident and I cleaned her up and gave her a shower. Then after that I got her breakfast ready and she was eating when Carrie came to put her make-up on, and set out her church clothes.

During these activities this week end, she has been less cooperative in all her activities. She has been more morose than in the past. I can tell that she is not doing as well as in the past. She is going down hill. Her condition moves from one level to another as it has in the past. She will probably stay in this level for several days or weeks, and then deteriorate a little more.

I am going to meet with a lady with a caregiving agency to find out how I can get some daily assistance. I am feeling more frustrated and depressed with her condition. I don't want my attitude toward Nell to get to where I become angry. Momentarily, I can get angry, (I guess more frustration and impatience) but I don't want that attitude to set in, or cause me to say unkind words.

7/13/2016   Nell usually goes to bed around 8:00 P.M. during this period of summer time. I don't want her going to bed when it is light outside. I went into the bedroom to get the bed covers down so she could get into bed, when it was time. I layed out her night gown, got her medicine and tooth brush ready for her. She was watching television in the living room. I heard a thud sound and ran out to see what the noise was.

It was Nell, who had fallen on the floor. She got up from her chair and lost her balance. She was just laying there waiting for me to help her. By God's grace, she had not broken anything. We had just heard this day, that Betty Russel, a 1953 classmate of Nell's from Murphy High School, had fallen and was in the Providence Hospital with a broken hip.

7/13/2016   Today is another day. I am taking Nell to the Orchid Spa to have her nails done. She enjoys that, although you couldn't tell by her expression. She is stoic in her manner in most things. My own manner at times becomes short with family members when they come across as negative in my caregiving. I know they mean well, but I get impatient with them as I am longsuffering with Nell. I know they have their lives filled with activities with their work and family, but after a difficult time with Nell, I feel alone in my caregiving. Maybe there is anger in my emotion. I don't think it is directed toward family members, certainly not toward Nell. I think that it is a feeling of somewhat helplessness in taking care of Nell. It seems to be my whole life, and I am not doing a good job with the caregiving. It is seven in the morning, and I am going to get Nell up, feed her, take her to the toilet, then shower and dress her. That is a chore to start the day. She is always so easy to help in these matters. I have to be alert in her toilet needs. I need to make sure she has a bowel movement before I shower and dress her, or I will have to do it all over again. Usually, after breakfast is best for her to go to the toilet.

It is now 5:30 P.M. and I am getting our evening meal, which consists of chicken soup and rice brought to us by our neighbor. We had a good lunch today. We ate at Wendy's; and the menu was a hamburger, french fries and a frostie. It was raining and thundering, so we just sat in the restaurant until the rain subsided. I ordered a coffee and I was drinking the coffee, when all of a sudden Nell got up and headed toward the door.

At first I thought she was going to the restroom, because it was raining outside. I got up to follow her, to make sure that she would be safe. She went out in the rain and stood by the rider's door waiting for me to come and unlock it and let her in. There she was just standing in the rain.

A neighbor brought a four-legged walker for Nell. When she gets out of her chair, she can use the walker until she gets her balance, then she can walk without the walker. She might use it to feel more secure. I will have to see how she does, and then we will have to work on the safe way to use the walker.

BEGINS TO USE A WALKER

7/14/2016   I title this diary, Nell's Journey. It is also, Bill's journey. But of course it is all the families' journey. Some members are more engaged than others. Carrie is the closest to us, so she is more engaged on a daily basis. If not personally present, she is nearer on the telephone. I try to keep in touch with her concerning our daily activities. There are times when I have been overwhelmed by the caregiving difficulties. I am tried and tested in so many ways. Mostly, little things, one after the other. The constant presence and awareness not to let her out of my presence, is demanding.Now to talk about my journey, sounds selfish, but I am thankful to be able to take Nell to E. A. Roberts, or I think I will have mental problems. Tomorrow, is Nell's birthday and E. A. Roberts is having a birthday party for Nell. I am bringing the cake to the party at 2:00 P. M. Tomorrow night I plan on taking her to Outback Restaurant for her 80th birthday. Although she has a difficult time eating out, it will probably be the last time she is able to celebrate her birthday out at a restaurant.

7/15/2016   Today is Nelda's birthday. Today is also another level in Nell's disease. Normally, I get Nell up and either shower and dress her, depending on our morning activities, then breakfast. Then take her to the toilet. And then I get her up and put her robe and slippers on her. Then she goes to the toilet and has a bowel movement and changes her Depends. Then she comes to breakfast, where I am waiting on her. This is the normal procedure.

This morning I got her up and put her robe and slippers on her, and took her to the toilet. I went to the kitchen to finish preparing breakfast and was waiting on her. When I went to get her, she pulled the lid up, dropped her Depends and sat on the toilet without pulling up her gown and robe. When I went to her and checked her out she had dropped her Depends, but messed in her gown and robe. When she got up, the mess dropped to the floor and not in the toilet. I had a big cleaning up and disinfecting problem to deal with, then I showered her. Fed her breakfast.

The reason I note this in the diary, is that now I know that I will have to pull her dress, or gown up when she goes to the toilet, I will have to continue doing it. . She has forgotten the sequence. And once I help her, she relies on me to do that particular sequence, so from that point on, I have to do it, or she may not get it right, and I will have to clean the mess. What ever I do to help her once, I have to continue doing it. It is the same in feeding her. If she feeds herself, it takes her a good hour to eat a little meal. If I am in a hurry, then I feed her. From that moment on I have had to do most of her feeding. I have helped her pull up her Depends, and now she will come out of the restroom, even in to a public place for me to pull up her Depends. So, this is becoming mostly a more intensive caregiving responsibility.

Left home about 11:30 A.M. to pick up a birthday cake at Rouses,and then went to Belks to buy a birthday dress. After we purchased her dress we left to go to Morrison's for lunch. I noticed that Nell had messed her pants while we were in Belks.

So we went to E.A. Roberts to clean her up, then ate lunch at Dew Drop Inn. We returned to E.A. Roberts after lunch for Nell's birthday party. I took pictures and Nell enjoyed the party. There were about 22 people there to enjoy her party and sing happy birthday. We returned home about 3:30 P.M. and I got Nell ready for her nap.

I will get her new dress on her and take her out tonight for a birthday dinner at Longhorn's or Outback.

We had a good meal in sharing a prime rib at Longhorn's Restaurant. We chose the right restaurant. When I tried to pay my bill with a gift card that Jonathan and Tara gave us for Father's day, the manager came and told us that another gentleman paid our bill. During the meal, I had to help Nell eat her steak and sweet potato. So when I went to the table and told the gentleman and his wife how we appreciated their kind act of paying our bill, the lady, Mrs. Jeff Rymes said they thought it was so nice the way I fed Nell her meal. She said, she hoped if that ever became necessary in her life, that her husband would treat her as good as I treated Nell with her meal.

When we got home, Nell had messed in her Depends, and I had to give her a shower to clean her up before she dressed for bed. All in all, Nell had a good birthday experience.

My granddaughter Blake Stone and great granddaughter Brooklyn came and spent the night with us before they planned on going to their condominium, Phoenix West, in Orange Beach on Saturday.

7/16/2016 We got up on Saturday morning and had a good breakfast of pancakes, bacon, and scrambled eggs. Each plate also had a dish of mixed fresh fruit. We plan to go to granddaughter Kim's house for a yard sale this morning (Sat.).

Today is a down day for Nell. I hope her condition doesn't stay at this level. She seemed to sleep deeper and longer last night. She has been weak, and unsteady today. Her mental awareness has been a little foggy. This is the first day, that she fell asleep, when she was waiting in the car in front of the grocery store while I got several items of food. The continued fogginess may have been because of the busyness of the great grandchildren being here at the house. I noticed that her hands were very shaky.

Nell got up from her chair and used the walker to go to the bedroom bathroom, to get ready for bed, about 8:00 P.M. I was cooking in the kitchen and did not notice that she had left the room. I went in to check on her and get her ready for bed. I sat on a bedroom chair and watched her brush her teeth and using the walker, she went to the side of her bed. I just watched from my chair to see if she could get into bed by herself. She got up on the side of the bed, but not far enough and slipped off the edge of the bed, and nearly falling on her back, grabbed on the sheets to hold herself, and I jumped up and caught her before she fell to the floor. She was very afraid that she might fall and hurt herself. I got her back in bed. I relate this story because it was the first time she used her walker from her chair to the bathroom and then attempted to use it to go get in bed.

7/25/2016   The last several days have been encouraging and discouraging. The discouraging things has been her weaknesses at times, her inability to comprehend what I say to her. She is weak at times in walking or getting in and out of her chair. The mental part is manifest in the way she ignores or the inability to process what I say, and she is unable to speak or reply. Then at other times it is encouraging that she can comprehend and complete a sentence in response to my question or statement. At times she seems to be "with" me, and other times she does not seem to be present.

Last night I had a difficult time getting Nell out of bed to go to the potty to empty her bladder. If I don't get her to the toilet in the middle of the night, then her Depends gets too full and the overflow wets the bed. I get her up and change her Depends and she may or may not need to empty her bladder at that time. When she got up last night she stepped on her bed stool as I was at her side to help her stand up. She was on the bed stool and her feet slipped forward and she slid down the bed. I tried to catch her with my sore right arm. We were at an impasse. She could not get traction on the floor to help support her body. I had all of her weight in my arms. I was unable to lift her with my painful right arm. I determined no matter the pain to lift her up so she could stand. I knew that if she got on the floor, I would need help to get her up. I could reach her walker and put it in position for her to push up with her arms on the walker to give me the help to get her upright.

I don't know what the future holds if I am unable to get Nell in and out of bed. I hate to think of a nursing home as has been suggested. Nell has a lovely, comfortable home that she has yearned to live in all of her life. I could not move her from her home. I am thinking now, on what to do to make arrangements for home care, or replace bedroom furniture in a way that I can get her up and down, and she can maneuver around so she can stay at home.

Last week, I made an appointment with Comfort Care to come to our house on Monday, to make an evaluation of Nell's needs. It was a good plan to make this appointment in light of the problem we had overnight in getting out of bed.

7/25/2016   Met with Comfort Care today to discuss caregiver assistance. I do not think there is any continuing help they have to offer, except a home health care nurse several times a month and someone to help Nell with physical therapy. I will have the therapist come to instruct us in several things to make it easier for me as a caregiver to get Nell in and out of bed.

After Nell took her nap today, she was not able to have a bowel movement in the toilet. She had an accident before she got to the toilet and I had a mess to clean up on her body, wash the bathroom carpets and mop the floor, not withstanding to clean the toilet.

I got her bathed and sat her down in her chair and looked into her eyes and told her not to worry about it. I told her I loved her. She just looked at me and tried to say something, but was unable to get it out, and she just choked up. I don't think she is capable of tearing up, but was very emotional and sorry about what happened, but she could not express her feelings. When I was mopping the bathroom floor and cleaning the carpet in our bedroom, my heart was warmed with the idea, that she is the mother of our children and has always been so faithful to God, humble in spirit and dedicated to her family. What's a little "mess!"

7/26/2016   Today began in a very difficult way. Nelda got up from bed with my help. I put her robe on her. She got into her slippers and I helped her to go to the toilet. As usual I then go into the kitchen to complete our breakfast menu. When she is through on the toilet she comes to the kitchen. I don't normally insist that she wears her Depends because as soon as she is through with breakfast I give her a shower and dress her.

She was a little longer than usual so I went back to see what her delay was in coming to breakfast. When I got to the bathroom, she had walked into the shower with her robe and slippers on and turned on the water. Her robe and slippers were soaken wet. She came to breakfast in her night gown and barefoot.

I was so worn out from that disappointed beginning. I started her in the shower and cleaned up all the mess. Then I dressed her and took her to E.A. Roberts for the day. I had the day to accomplish a few tasks at home

I fixed dinner tonight. I finished and went into the other room while Nell continued her dinner. I heard a thud! She fell off her chair and hit the edge of a corner of the wall in the breakfast area. She hit so hard, I thought it necessary to take her to the emergency for a ct scan. I took her to Mobile Infirmary and after the test, they said she was not bleeding. She had a high blood pressure. I gave her another bp medicine when I got her home. Her bp was 188/82.

I felt so disturbed about Nell's needs today that I had thoughts about having her reside in a Nursing Home. I could not have that happen again. Maybe it is not possible to care for her at home. I was at my wit's end. But she would have to be in a Memory Care ward and that costs about $3-4,000.00 a month, which would be out of the question. A home caregiver costs $15.00 per hour. I have resigned myself to the idea of being more attentive.

7/28/2016   Comfort care sent three caregivers to my house today to minister to Nell. The first one was an occupational therapist. Not quite sure the help she gave was needed. The next one was a physical therapist. She did some exercises, such as walking and turning in a circle. She got her in and out of bed and up and down on the commode. All of that was good and what she did all the time. She watched and coached her get up from her sofa chair to begin walking with a walker with wheels. She said she needed to strengthen her legs. I realize that to strengthen her legs takes a number of visits per week, over a long period of time. I was not in favor of that kind of a schedule. I take Nell to the Y, and walk her up and down the street for a regular exercise. We walk around WalMart also. I was not convinced that I needed to adjust my schedule to have the therapist come on a regular basis, so I told her not to come. I Would see that she got exercise, which I did. We would go to the Y in Saraland for Nell to ride the exercise bicycle. She would ride it slow, but, at least, she was exercising.

7/28/2016   A friend is coming to be with Nell today, in a lady's day out activity of shopping and lunch. That is not easy. I pray that all goes well. She seems to be doing well after her fall Tuesday night. I gave her a cup of coffee in her chair this morning and she dropped off to sleep and spilled the whole cup of coffee in her lap.

A friend took Nell shopping and had lunch at Steak & Shake. She was home about 2:00 PM. My son-in-law Calvin and I took the box springs from our bed, which lowered the mattress about 8 inches. Nell went into the bedroom to take a nap, and she looked mixed up, and confused. But she jumped right on the bed and took a nap. When she got up, she seemed to be more confortable with the walker. She just carried it in front of her. She used it for security in her walking. When she went to bed, she jumped right in easily, rather than stepping on her bed stool and struggle to get in bed as was the case with the higher bed.

7/30/2016   We had a long day this Saturday. We left our house to pick up Dexter from Serenity Care at Grelot and

Dawes Rd. so he could come to our house and do yard work. Nell and I drove again out to Hillcrest Baptist Church to attend the funeral of a friend. Later in the day I took Dexter home and then stopped at the Golden Corral on Schillinger Rd in West Mobile for dinner. I noticed that Nell was not as alert, she would hardly respond at times to me as I tried to feed her. She is almost to the place where she is unable to feed herself. She gets so shaky with her utinsels that she cannot get them to her mouth. She is also so weak in her legs that I have to keep my eyes and hands on her when she is on her feet. If she is sitting down, she will get up if she can, from whatever she is sitting on and her first few steps are very erratic. She was so tired when we got home tonight from dinner, that I got her ready to get in bed. In just a few moments she was asleep. Today was a busy day, also a day in which I noticed a drop off in her ability to recognize and listen to me.

I got an application from Little Sisters of the Poor. I would like Nell to go there if something happened to me and I was unable to care for her. They have such a long waiting list, that I thought I would be prepared and then the transition from home to their Memory Care Unit would not be so difficult. She would have to pay the $3,000.00 plus for the first month and then the following months would be taken care of by Medicare, according to our social worker from Comfort Care. I will get more information on this.

8/11/2016 Nell and I drove to Huntsville on the 2nd of August, and she stayed with daughter Kimberly, while I flew to Columbus, Ohio. I was honored to officiate at grandson Will Whitfield IV wedding to Bethany Cruise. Nell was not able to travel to Columbus and stay around those few days of wedding rehearsal and the wedding on Friday night, so I flew by myself. I flew back to Huntsville, on Saturday. We returned to Saraland on Sunday. Nell's few days with Kim were very good. Nell was painting her lake house and Nell had her walker with wheels, and walked around a lot. Since she got the walker with wheels she has moved around a lot more and, in a sense, she has got more independent in her movements.

She has been a lot more conscious of her bathroom habits, especially her bowel movements. That is, she has gone to the bathroom when she has felt the urge.

When we came home about 12:30 PM, I fed her and she then took a nap. After her nap, we went for a walk to the end of the street. She did very good with her walker with wheels. She has a tendency to lean a little too much and starts to walk too fast as we go down the street incline. I have to hold on to the walker. When we got to the front door, she began to fall because of her weak, tired legs as she tried to lift the walker up the front steps.

Last week in Huntsville, Nell had a bladder infection. I called the doctor in Mobile and he sent a prescription to Walgreens in Huntsville, and I picked it up on Saturday. She has been feeling so much more alert since she has been taking it. She doesn't appear to have the infection today, Thursday, Aug. 11. But Carrie said to continue the dosage a few more days.

Yesterday, an unusual thing happened. I put Nell down for a nap about 2:00 PM. I was working in the kitchen, when I heard her call to me. It was plain, and it was how she calls, "Bill". I was startled and I immediately went back to the bedroom thinking she fell out of the bed and was laying on the floor. As I was going back to the bedroom, I heard her call again, "Bill." When I opened the door I was pleased to see her laying on her stomach sound asleep. I don't think she called in that position, even in her sleep. I think I just heard her call, in my imagination. But it was so real, and the inflection was just like she calls to me. I don't feel bad, or stressful, or in any way mentally or emotional unbalanced, as far as I know, to hear a call like this in my imagination.

8/30/2016   I have not made any notes for some time. There were several things that have happened to cause me to write some new notes. We went to Huntsville, where Nell stayed for several days, while I flew to Columbus, Ohio to officiate at Will's wedding to Bethany. We also went to the Gulf for several days to play golf and shop with the friends. All went well with Nell.

When we returned, she had a urinary tract infection. I had a bad cold. After we went to Urgent Care and got prescriptions to help the healing process, all went well, after 4 or 5 days.

Nell complained of not feeling well on Monday, and seemed depressed. She did not look at me with a good disposition. I asked if she was angry with me? She said: "angry with you." I asked her why? She did not answer. We had an appointment with our primary physician, Dr. Whetstone on Monday. He said her urine sample taken that morning was clear. He said mine had blood in it, and he made an immediate appointment for me with Dr. Oswalt, for the next day, I think Nell was aware of what Dr. Whetstone said to me, and Nell understood this was not good, and she got depressed, wondering if something happened to me, who would take care of her. That is a concern of mine, and I know a concern of God, so I have put it in His hands. I have filled out application to Little Sisters of the Poor, and hopefully be able to have her accepted there as a resident, if I was unable to care for her.

8/31/6   I completed the application to Little Sisters of the Poor memory care unit, except submitting the last six months of Nell's checking account and her prescriptions she takes and took them to the Little Sisters and today I mailed those additional items listed above. I have been concerned about two things for the reason to get my application for Nell to the Little Sisters. The first is that Nell is getting more difficult for me to care for her. She is getting where she can hardly walk. It is getting more difficult for Nell to eat. She cannot go to the restroom by herself. In a public restroom, someone has to go in with her or I have to go in when it is empty and help her and make sure her Depends is OK, and we can get them up before she exits the Women's room. If I wait, she comes out and says she needs help. If she has a bowel movement in the restroom, then I have to clean her.

I gave her a bowl of ice cream after supper tonight. She could not eat the balance of ice cream and got up and came to me for help to put the ice cream on her spoon and put it in her mouth, so she could eat it.

The second reason I felt I had to make application to Little Sisters, is because I have been having health problems which gave me concern that if I was unable to take care of Nell, then she would need to go into a nursing home. I would rather have her at Little Sisters.

We had an appointment with Nell's neurologist today. We were asked to schedule another for six months from today. I didn't schedule another appointment. The neurologist nor any other doctor can help Nell in her Alzheimer's disease. He asked Nell, "How is your family?" She asked him "How is your family?" Dr Hecker asked again, "How is YOUR family?" She did not respond. Dr. Hecker was compassionate in his concern, but you could tell that there was nothing he could do. I may not make another appointment with a doctor except our primary doctor.

About 6:30 P.M., Nell got up from her chair and went to the bedroom. I did not know she left the room. When I went in to the bedroom she was laying on the bed. I got her up and got the toothbrush ready and her pill to take, then got her bed ready and put her to bed. When I went to the bathroom she was just playing with the sink with her toothbrush. I had to put the toothbrush into her mouth. She brushed a little then began washing her toothbrush. It appears that if she is going to have her teeth brushed, I will have to do that. She cannot mentally handle that chore, any more than eat or pull up her Depends. It is getting, really, that I have to take her to the toilet and pull her Depends down and sit her rightly on the commode. Then pull up her Depends and her dress.

9/1/2016   This morning while we were having breakfast, Nell indicated she needed to go to the toilet, which I help her to go to "potty". After she got up from the commode, (which she didn't do anything: she thought it was time to go to bed and went to pull the covers down. I took her hand to lead her back to the patio and finish her breakfast. This is the kind of confusion that she exhibits during the day. She is mixed up concerning a lot of things. She is now sitting in her chair sleeping. It is 10:30 A.M.

9/2/2016   When Nell was diagnosed with Alzheimer's disease, I tried to talk to individuals and read various articles on Alzheimer disease, and did not find anything that spoke to Nell's symptoms. It seems that each individual is different. I decided to write some accounts of my experience. For instance, I took her to Urgent Care where they diagnosed Nell with a UTI. After she took medicine for several days which caused diarhea, they called and said that tests came back and she did not have a UTI. I followed up with our primary physician and he said she had a UTI, but would not prescribe medicine until a culture informed him of the type of UTI. I could not take her to E.A. Roberts because the doctor said she had a UTI. I needed to take her to E.A. Roberts on Friday morning because I was scheduled for c-scan due to bleeding in my kidney. On Thursday night I got a call that the culture came back and she did not have a UTI. I took her to E.A. Roberts on Friday morning early and she had not had a bowel movement as yet. I did not return to pick her up until about 5:45 P.M. I took advantage of this time to work on my homecoming message at Cypress Shores Baptist Church on September 11. Also, I filled out papers from the V.A. to apply for help costs for Nell as a veteran's wife. I had to take that to my primary physician, for him to sign. When I went to pick Nell up from E.A. Roberts, the nurse told me that she had a terrible rash on her genital area. I asked her to show me. When she pulled down her Depends, she was wet and somewhat dirty, which was unusual for E. A. Roberts. I stopped at Walgreen's drug store in Saraland and asked the druggist what I needed to put on her rash. I purchased that and when we arrived home, I gave her a shower and cleaned and dried the genital area. The rash was a horrible red! It was difficult to see and may have been there when I showered her in the morning, because as I tried to wash her when I got her home, I had to look under her bottom to see it. Just soaping and rinsing I could not see it. It may have been there several days.

I got to thinking about the reason she had been standing up from the table or from the chairs when we went somewhere, that she could have been hurting for several days. She even sat on the front of her chair to eat and would lean over and the chair went back. I just thought she was unsettled. I would push the chair back up. And she would go through the same routine. That may even be a reason that she said a day or so earlier that she didn't like me. It could be that she was hurting and was unable to tell me, but she wanted help, and I would not help her.

I tell this story graphically, to relate this to any Alzheimer caregiver to look over your patient thoroughly day to day in every way. Today, she pulled her right hand away from me indicating pain in some way. I asked if she hurt her wrist, and she replied, "Hurt." I don't know when she hurt it. I think I would have known.

I have applied for a memory care residence at Little Sisters of the Poor, because if something happened to me, Nell would need to go to a Nursing Home. It is very hard to get into the Little Sisters, and I thought if her name came up, and we were not at that point yet, I could drop down for a later day. But the lady phoned me today and said they had a room for Nell. I had to tell her, I was not ready. Later I called the social worker at Little Sisters, that I needed to consult with my children about this. I left her a message, and she has not called me back. I do not know at this time if I need to have surgery for my bleeding kidney, then I would need help with Nell for that time and recuperating period, so I wanted to talk to the social worker about my situation, and I could not get an answer from my urologist until after Labor Day.

9/5/2016 This is Labor Day, and this is the fourth day since I have been aware of Nell's rash. The irritation does not seem as bad as when first discovered, but it is still very red in places. This has been a trying weekend, full of worries for Nell's condition. Not knowing what to do is the worry. I called my neighbor on Saturday evening. She worked in the Mobile Infirmary Emergency, and now works in the cardiac department at Springhill. I explained the situation and she did not think it was an emergency as long as I was putting the medicine on her rash and it seemed to be getting better. I will take Nell to her doctor Tuesday or Nell's gynecologist.

The most difficult part in my caregiving is to question myself if I am doing what is best for Nell, when she has a physical, mental or emotional problem, where if she was in a nursing home facility, they have trained nurses and most times the caregivers at the facility have experienced these things before and know what to do.

9/9/2016   I took Nell to E A Roberts today, and I played golf with some men from the church. I bathed Nell and fixed and fed her breakfast before we left to E. A. Roberts. I took her to the toilet before we left and she had an accident in her Depends. I had to give her a shower, apply medicine again on her rash, put fresh Depends on her, and then help her in the car to leave.

The last week, Nell has been very slow to respond, and seemingly less able to relate to her environment. I am overwhelmed sometimes with the constant care Nell needs. I cannot let her get out of my sight, for fear she will fall. She gets tired easily, and wants to go to bed early, like 6:00 P.M. I try to delay until 7:00 P.M. It is more difficult to go out to eat. It is easier to get "take out" meals and let her try to eat at home. It takes a long time for her to eat if we eat in a restaurant. I have to get her up from sleep during the night several times because I don't want wet Depends with her rash.

9/10/2016   This Saturday morning Nell has been very sleepy. After breakfast she sat in her chair and went to sleep. Later, when we went to meet granddaughter Stacey for lunch at the Blue Gill Restaurant, she was sleepy as we drove, which she usually stays awake and alert while riding in the car. When we got home she went right in to her bedroom to take a nap. I don't know if the rash is causing her tiredness. This tiredness is unusual. I just can't believe this tiredness is only caused by her Alzheimer's.

9/14/2016   We went to Primetimers on Monday for lunch and entertainment. Nell had to be fed. She fell asleep during the entertainment, and had an accident in her Depends during the entertainment. I went to the lady's room to clean her with the help of a retired nurse who is a member of our church. When we got home, she took a nap. I generally let her sleep for about an hour and a half. Then that evening about 6:00 P.M. she went to the bedroom to go to bed. I thought this tiredness was due to her having the rash, and daughter Carrie thought it might be shingles. I made a doctor's appointment and was able to see the doctor on Wednesday (today). The doctor said her rash was not shingles, but like jock itch or athletes's foot kind of rash. He prescribed a medicine to take orally and advised me to continue the medicine to rub on her rash twice a day. Nell is unable to do anything in a good way for herself. If she tries to eat, she drops the food from her utinsel on her clothes. She can't dress or undress herself. She can't shower herself nor dry herself. She needs assistance to go to the bathroom. She can't brush her teeth.

9/25/2016   It has been awhile since I added any comments. Friday, I went to Dr. Coleman Oswalt for a bladder infection and took Nell with me. When we went into the examining room Nell came with me and sat in a chair and had an accident while we were waiting. I had to wait to clean her when we went home. This was the second time she did this in the waiting room with Dr. Oswalt.

The first time I cleaned her up in the waiting room toilet area. Not this time! There was no sink, it just had a toilet. After I noticed she had an accident, I held her and said, "I love you." She responded to me with a bunch of jumbled words as she looked at me with an affectionate look. I kind of knew what she was trying to say. When we got home, I showered her and put medicine on the rash, as I do in the morning and night.

The rash, I have mentioned in the above notes is getting a lot better.

Last night Nell got up in the middle of the night and went to the toilet. I was asleep and didn't hear her until she was getting back in bed. She was stuck and couldn't make it. I thought she was just getting out of bed, so I got up and took her to the bathroom and noticed her Depends on the floor in front of the toilet. So that is when I understood she had already gotten up and when I discovered her she had already gone to the toilet and was coming back to bed. So unusual. I normally get her up and take her to the toilet in the middle of the night. So I put some new Depends on her and put her to bed. In the morning I got up about 5:00 A.M., and was reading on the back patio. About 7:00 A.M., the usual time I get her up and feed her breakfast, she got up by herself and came out to the back patio. I let her sit there and brought her breakfast to her on the back patio.

I didn't take Nell to worship services this morning, which is the second Sunday she missed, because she goes to sleep and after the services a number of times I have taken her to the Lady's restroom and the church ladies have had to clean her, so in order to maintain her dignity, I decided this was best, especially not to take Nell to worship services today, especially, after we had attended a luncheon at church with the seniors on Monday, which was embarrassing for her. I had to feed her and when I went to the restroom with her before we left, I had to clean her and put on new Depends with the help of one of the ladies from the church. I did not feel it was good for her dignity.

Last Sunday, my daughter Carrie stayed with Nell, while I went to church. She attended her worship services then rushed to meet me by her church to pick up Nell and stay with her until

I returned. This Sunday, Bill came from Gulfport, Ms., area to stay with Nell. I am trying to get a lady to come in on Sundays, and Wednesdays for several hours, while I attend church activities in which I participate.

9/28/2016   Today, was a difficult day for me. I had a sitter come to be with Nell while I attended the Senior Choir rehearsal. Nell usually comes to rehearsal and sings. She has done so good at singing all the old Christian hymns and songs. Most of the hymns she knew by heart. But at the last rehearsal she just slept and dropped her depends in the choir room to get ready to go to the toilet. Some around her were amused. I was embarrassed for her. I took her to the women's restroom.

I didn't want to continue to damage her image and dignity, so decided not to take her to rehearsal today. While singing one of her favorite songs, I got emotional and choked up and tears came to my eyes. No one around me noticed. I kept to myself. The reason I became so emotional was because of an incident that happened right after I became a Christian. We were singing in church, and Nell was so full of joy, that her husband had become a Christian and was sitting beside her in church and singing about the Jesus that she loved and was so faithful to her for so many years. After church in a casual way, I said, "You know when you sing, often you just get louder, rather than go up a note, and sing softer, when you go down a note." After that, Nell was very timid with her singing. Sometimes I would say, "Let's see if we can sing this certain song together." She would say, "You know I can't sing." She could sing, but because of my remark for all the 62 years of marriage (At least from the time I became a Christian), Nell would not sing with me, because of the remark I made. I would say, "You can sing Nell, come on, let's sing together." "No," she would say, "I can't sing." So, through the many years, even as the wife of the pastor, she would sing in church, but not with me. I sang in the choir where I was pastor, when it was convenient. The choir director asked Nell to sing in the choir, and she declined. Never did she sing in the choir, until we began to sing in the senior choir. Other choir members would ask her why she didn't sing in the choir, and she would remark that, our choir director would not even want her to pray for the choir. She always got a laugh with others for that remark, and they would say, that was not so.

This morning as I was rehearsing with the senior choir, others asked where Nell was? I told them that Nell was with a sitter. While I was singing, it came to my mind that I had told Nell right after I became a Christian, that she did not follow the notes, implying she could not sing good. She did not sing with the joy she had in singing after that. It went for all these years like that up until these last several years when we sang together in the senior choir. But, this morning, she was not here with me singing in the senior choir, and I became so emotional with the hurt that I caused in her heart over saying that about her singing. Yet, she was always so kind and casual about it. I was so choked up about my careless remark so many years ago, and here I was so emotionally choked up, because I could not relate to her about that now. It was back in the past. I could think about it, but I don't think she is capable of thinking about it now.

9/29/2016   The last two nights, Nell has got up by herself. The night before last, she was half way out of bed, and when I went to the toilet I noticed that she had already gone to the toilet and left her Depends on the floor. So, I determined she was half way into bed. I had to put on a dry Depends and helped her back in bed. Last night, I got up about 3:00 A.M., to go to the toilet. When I was returning to bed, I met her about half way to the toilet. I helped her go to the toilet, and then put on a dry Depends and helped her back to bed. Both nights were unusual. This afternoon, she went back to her bedroom to take a second nap. This was about 4:00 PM. I went to the kitchen to prepare our evening meal. After about 30 minutes I went to wake her up and she was sitting on the toilet. I was surprised, because she hadn't done this lately.

THE BEGINNING OF A HELPING AGENCY

The Therapist from Kindred Care came today and examined Nell. She said Nell had a sore shoulder. Nell followed several of her commands, and her right shoulder was not responding well. She thought she might have had a stroke, but with further exercises, she decided I should have her see our orthopedic doctor for a sore shoulder. I made an appointment with him on Friday to have him look it over, xray, or what ever needs to be done.

We went to have the orthopedist xray the shoulder and he said there was no problem, most likely, pulled muscle or cartilege. He gave her a shot in the shoulder, and gave me a slip to give to the therapist so she could continue treating Nell with some physical therapy. After several days of observing, I think she had a small stroke and her right arm is not responding as it should.

10/5/2016   Yesterday, Nell had a hard time getting up in the morning after a night's sleep. She stood up, closed her eyes and tried to continue her sleep. I showered her and gave her breakfast, then dressed her. She sat down while I cleaned up the Kitchen and made the bedroom and picked up the bathroom. Nell just slept. She tried to sleep many times during the day. That was yesterday, today, is different. She is more alert, but her demeanor is very subdued. She just got up from her nap, about 4:00 P.M., and has eaten a snack of jello. She layed her head back on the chair and closed her eyes, for about 2 minutes and now opened her eyes and looked around. She is very restless; she keeps getting up and standing, then sitting. I don't know what to do, she can't tell me or give me a clue.

10/6/2016 This morning after breakfast, Nell sat out on the back patio, while I cleaned up the kitchen and bedroom. I sat with her for awhile, and played some Pandora Christian music. She likes that, but seemed to go off to sleep. After about 15 minutes I woke her up and asked her if she wanted to sit on the front porch and wait for Netta. Netta was coming today, while I went to see my neurologist. When we got inside the house, I had her stand just inside the patio door, while I placed some dishes on the bar. She lost her balance and fell backwards against the patio door and sat hard on the floor. When I helped her up she seemed to give way to her left leg while walking to her chair. As she sat on her chair, I checked her leg, she seemed ok, so we continued on to sit on the front porch. Earlier in the morning, after I got her dressed, I asked her to sit on the bathtub edge, while I put her shoes on her. She sat down, but not far enough and slipped down on the floor and fell back and hit her head on the door jam of the closet. She didn't hit hard, but it frightened both of us. She has been more wobbly these last few days. I don't know if this is a permanent stage.

10/8/2016 This is Saturday morning, looking back over this past week, my read is that Nell's condition has deteriorated somewhat. She is so unsteady on her feet, she fell twice. I took my hand off of her for a second or two, and she lost her balance and fell. Luckily it was close to a wall so she fell into the wall (patio doors), and it was not a hard fall. But she has had some shakes these past three days. Her right arm is indicating a partial stroke, I believe, rather than an injury.

I don't know if Nell knows who I am at this stage. I believe she recognizes me as the one who is taking care of her, much like the caregivers at E.A. Roberts. When she is in bed, she will roll over towards me and put her arm around me, much like she did when she was her normal self.

Something that has concerned me, is that when she gets out of the shower, her nose will run. Also, when I feed her, it runs. It may be a result of stress. It doesn't last long. No matter where I feed her, in a restaurant, or at home, it is the same. It seems if I let her piddle in feeding herself, her nose does not run, it runs when I begin to feed her. There may be exceptions, but that is the general experience.

Saturday, at 10:30 AM, we attended the open house of the opening of the new gymnasium at Dauphin Way Baptist Church. We had to return home after about a half hour because Nell had an accident. We came home and I cleaned her up and put new clothes on her bottom part. She just stands while I clean her and it looks like she shows no remorse. She just stands still. I told her, "I love you." She responded in a few words of gibberish. I think it was asking for forgiveness or something like being sorry for the accident.

10/9/2016 Wynetta came today to sit with Nell, while I attended worship services at Dauphin Way Baptist. I had a pork roast in the slow cooker along with vegetables. Wynettta had it all ready when I came home for Sunday Dinner. We ate, she cleaned up the kitchen and left to go home. Nell ate good and seemed to get along well with Wynetta. Wynetta got her dressed and took care of her while I was gone.

One of the experiences of being a caregiver is to have the therapists and nurses come to our home to do what they are instructed to do with the patient. Of course the most often they come the more they get paid. They want to come at their convenience, and sometimes that does not work for our schedule. I finally said that Mondays and Thursdays would be best for us but to phone before coming. That seems to work but the nurse will have someone else call to come and give a bath or do occupational therapy. If I don't think Nell needs what they do at that time I don't make an appointment.

I am with Nell 24/7, and I don't need activity and intrusion that makes my caregiving more difficult. For instance, if we plan on going somewhere, and just as we are leaving, they call because they are in the area. But if I don't see a need for their services at that time, I tell them we will not be home at that time.

10/11/2016   I took Nell to E.A. Roberts today, while I played golf at Magnolia Grove Golf Course with several men from Dauphin Way Baptist. I picked her up around 3:30 P.M.after the golf game and we went to Orchid Day Spa to get pedicures. Nell seemed very tired and could hardly walk. She was very shaky and unstable. I had to keep her very close to me, because I was concerned about her falling. After the pedicure we went home and had supper. She went right to bed. She hardly spoke since she came home from E. A. Roberts. Usually, she would respond by repeating what I would say to her, but today she responded very little.

10/12/2016   Yesterday, when I picked Nell up at E.A. Roberts, she seemed to be quite tired and unsteady on her feet. I had a more difficult time getting her awake and up this morning. She was lethargic. I fed her breakfast and waited for the caregiver to come and give her a bath. She did not show up. Wynetta came at 10:00 A.M., and gave her a shower. I left at 10 to rehearse with our Senior Choir. Afterwards I had a lunch by myself. It was good to eat without taking into consideration feeding Nell. When I returned about 1:30 P.M., Wynetta had fed Nell from the meals we received from "Meals on Wheels." She had layed her on the bed for a nap, before she left. When I awakened her about an hour and a half later, it was difficult getting her to stand up and walk. We went to the grocery store. Nell pushed her walker and I placed a box on the walker seat to put groceries into it. That way, I got Nell to walk. She had a hard time with the walker. She would lean forward and walk faster and faster, and I would have to keep my hand on her and the walker because I was concerned she might fall face down on the tile. My comment about her day would be that she was very lethargic, unsteady, very little words, and sleepy, like drugged sleepy. Hope she picks up tomorrow.

10/12/2016   Today, my emotions were up and down. This morning I was pleased with Nell. I decided not to make breakfast but to go to Hardees. She ate a Sausage/biscuit and tator tots, all by herself. She drank her orange juice. We went to WalMart and did some grocery shopping. She sat in a rolling chair with a basket where I could put groceries. We came home and she went to the toilet. I fed her lunch and then she took her usual nap from about 1-2:30 P.M. She watched a little football, I took her for a walk with her walker, and then I gave her supper. All during the day she said very little. Usually, I can get her to repeat something, but not today. After supper I took her to get ready for bed. It was about 6:00 PM. When I took her clothes off, I discovered that she had a accident in her Depends. I had to clean her in the shower and dress her for bed.

Tonight was the first time I could say, that I was very upset with Nell. Even knowing she cannot help what she does, and has no ability to talk, or get a thought expressed, I was upset with her. I think, a lot of my anger was that she does not talk to me in all that I am doing for her, and then has and accident in her Depends, and I have to bear the smell and the mess, clean her up with no evident response. There is no one around to give a word of encouragement, and this lonliness is also desire to follow my Covenant Prayer.

Sometimes when I go to wake Nell up in the morning or from a nap, and I cannot tell if she is breathing. I hate to even admit that a thought comes into my mind, that maybe she has died. I almost hope that is the case, but then a horrible thought comes into my mind, that I would even think like that. I don't feel guilty about my thought, because I think that her death would be best for her, our family and myself. Still, I want to do all I can to keep her well and alive, as long as God in His Providence wills it, and I take the responsibility seriously, to care for Nell as long as He wills it. I may have to take her to a nursing home sometime in the future, but I think that would be harder for me to go regularly every day and feed her and tend to her there. This is my life now, to take care of Nell. I will do the best I can. I feel I can do better care at home than in a nursing home.

10/13/2016   Today, Wynetta came to be with Nell while I went to church. I also went to lunch after church services with friends. I came home and put Nell on the bed for her afternoon nap. Wynetta left. After I got her up from her nap, I noticed she had some blood in her Depends. Later we went to my daughter Carrie's home for the evening meal. When we got back around 6:00 P.M. I changed her depends and there was blood on the Depends. When she dried herself there was blood on the toilet tissue. It was not a lot of blood, just evidences of blood. I asked her does your stomach ache, and she replied: "Stomach aches." She does repeat things I say, but I don't think she would have repeated those words, unless her stomach really ached. I am going to get an appointment with the doctor in the morning. She seemed to have a good attitude most of the time I was with her today. She still is a little wobbly and weak. Her balance is not good either. I asked her if she was tired when I put her to bed. She said, "Tired."

I have a better temperament today regarding Nell. I am so sorry for my bad feelings at times I have toward her. Later when I feel better, I feel bad for the anger if I may describe the feelings in that manner. Especially tonight with the blood issue, I really feel bad about myself. I feel a tender love toward Nell.

11/2/2016   It has been awhile since I added any comments because my laptop was being repaired. It seems to be working now. Several weeks ago, Nell got up from bed, about 2:00 A.M. I reached over during the night and she was not there. I got up and went to see if she went to the toilet. She was not there, so I went to the living room. I saw the garage door open and Nell was laying on the floor with her arm holding up her head. She was very cold. I don't know how long she was there, for she does not call out. Not that she is incapable, but she does not initiate any conversation. About a week later, she fell out of bed. I was asleep and heard a "thump" and it waked me up. I felt her side of the bed, and she was gone. I got up and went around the bed and there she was laying on the floor.

Yesterday morning I went through my regular routine of getting Nell up. When I removed her Depends, I helped her get on the toilet. She sat there for several minutes, and came to take a shower, and had an accident on the way. I got her into the shower. I had to clean the floor from the accident. I mention this because this is a caregiver experience when you are caring for a loved one who has Alzheimer's. As I was rinsing her off, I got to thinking, most partners would let the nursing home handle all of the messes. I have had to clean her up in church, in restaurants, in a pedicure salon, in a service station restroom, in the waiting room of a doctor's office, in an airline waiting room, at the movies and other places. Most partners would give up on all that and let a nursing home do all the cleaning up. I am handling it up to now. I am glad she is active and I can go places with her. Who knows what tomorrow may bring. My children are ok with what I determine to be best.

Not only that, but the feeding, and taking care of her all day trying to keep her active and not sitting and sleeping is part of the caregiver responsibilities. All of that caring with no conversation because Nell is not able to get a thought together. I don't know what she wants to eat, or what she wants to watch on TV. It is difficult to take her to a restaurant to eat, because I have to feed her while I am trying to eat also. Today, I took her to her 1953 Murphy H.S. reunion at a restaurant. She was not able to relate, or converse with her classmates. I had to feed her. I didn't like it for her, but her caregiver who would come to relieve me for a few hours for events like this, didn't show up. This was the last time she attended a Murphy class reunion.

I took her to a movie on our 62 nd anniversary on October 23, 2016 and out to eat afterwards at Steak and Shake. I had to feed her and afterwards when I went to pay, a young man about 25 with his baseball hat on backwards, asked how long we had been married. He and his girl friend sat a couple of booths from us, and watched me feed Nell. I told him that she pinned my wings on me as a Marine pilot, and on this day 62 years ago, we got married. He said, "Thank you for your service, sir. Let me pay your check." I thought this to be kind and unusual for a man of his age to be so patriotic and polite to pay the check. He must have seen this in acts of his father.

11/5/2016 Saturday. We have been to the Alzheimer's walk this morning, and then did some chores to get my iPhone working. We had lunch at Morrisons then came home. Nell waited in the car for at least two hours in front of Verizon while I was getting help to replace a broken iphone. I could see her at all times, but I know that it was hard on her. She has been very down from the time she got up this morning until time to go to bed. I am very concerned about her physical and mental condition today. This morning (Sat) breakfast, she acted as if she was mad at me, and did not speak or respond to questions as she usually does (As limited as that is). That attitude seemed to be her attitude all day long.

11/7/206   Monday morning. I have been very concerned about Nell's condition. She has been unable to walk without help. If I took my hands off of her she would start falling. She was very slow on her feet, even with the walker. She had an accident on the bathroom rugs while Wynetta was taking her to the toilet, when I was in worship Sunday. Wynetta told me that she had to give her a shower, and throw the floor rugs into the washer. She brought Nell to meet me at Church, and Nell and I went to lunch at Morrisons with church friends. It was difficult as I fed her, and a number of Dauphin Way Baptist members and other friends saw her, and Nell had a scowl on her face, which caused the friends and members some concern. We came home and Nell took a nap. I gave her a snack afterwards on the back patio. I tried to engage her in conversation. I would mention the children's names and she would just stare at me, like I was a stranger, and then turn her face away from me. I don't think she knew me. There was a barrier between her and me. I tried to talk about things in her past, and she looked at me with hostility. I think this was the first time that I could say, that she showed no knowledge of who I was. When I put her to bed, I leaned over to give her a kiss and said, "I love you," and she responded, "I love you." I think she would say that to anyone, and she would parrot back what was said. I hold to the hope that she knew she was saying it to me.

This is 3:30 A.M., I got up because, I couldn't sleep. We will be facing another day. I have hopes that there would be a change in Nell's disposition. Or, it may be that this is just another permanent change. I am just about out of her depression medicine, and I don't think I will fill the prescription again. I don't think there is any help in it. I am even considering discontinuing giving her Donepezal, also. At one of the Alzheimer conferences, a doctor mentioned that there is a time when the medicine begins to have a big drop as to its effectiveness. I don't think there is any benefits to this medicine.

11/9/2016   Today has been a better day for Nell. Nell is walking, but very unsteady. She got up from bed more alert, mentally & physically and less wobbly. After she ate breakfast and I got her showered and dressed she sat out on the front porch. Soon she got up and I hovered over her to see where she would go. She went to the toilet. I had to clean her and help pull up her Depends and pants. After lunch, she layed down to take a nap.

11/27/2016   It has been several weeks since I have tried to type any comments on my caregiving. The laptop is so temperamental, I do not want to try it. Nell had a bladder infection about two weeks ago. I took her to her gynecologist. He examined her and determined it was a bladder infection. When she has a bladder infection her personality changes to a negative, and difficult personna. I understand. Especially after the diagnosis.

11/28/2016   The last few days I have been angry at times. Nell will not feed herself. When I feed her, she gets a running nose. I wipe, then feed. Wipe then give her a bite. Wipe and give another bite. Her nose does not run at any other time except when she eats and when I give her a shower. She is fine, then when she comes out of the shower, and I am drying her, she gets a runny nose. When you do this day after day, it is hard for me to keep a good attitude, especially when she turns her face away from me.

Last nite and this morning, she seemed to be angry with me. I told her that I loved her. I did all that I could do to see that she was well taken care of because I loved her. She would not speak a word, although that is all she can do, is speak a word. When I tell her I love her, she replies, "I love you." But last night and this morning she said not a word. All day she appeared to be angry.

11/29/2016   Last night Nell's nephew, sent me a message that his dad, Nell's brother in law, died in Tuscaloosa. It was about 8:00 PM., and I decided to wait and inform her this morning. While I was giving her a shower I told her that Fred died. She did not make any kind of response. I told her several times during breakfast that Fred died. I said, "Fred was your sister Julia's husband." She did not even comprehend about the mention of her sister's name. The funeral is day after tomorrow (Thursday), in Tuscaloosa. I will drive up to represent Nell at the funeral of her sister's husband. I took her to E.A. Roberts today, and picked her up about 4:00 PM. There was no difference in her demeanor, nor her emotions. I put her to bed tonight, and there was no acknowledgement in any manner that her sister's husband died. So, I will leave her at E. A. Roberts and drive up myself to represent Nell at her sister's funeral.

I drove up to the funeral in Tuscaloosa. After the funeral Ike had to go back to his law practice, and Nell's cousin in law Carole (Ike's wife)and her grandaughter, Emily were kind enough to take me to lunch. Nell's in-laws did not invite us to participate in their family meal at the Holy Spirit Catholic Church. Nell's cousin Ike and wife Carol were quite close to Nell's brother in law, after Nell's sister, Julia died several years ago.

12/7/2016   This past week Nell has been more distant and unresponsive to any kind of relationship to me. It is like being a stranger in my own house with my wife of 62 years. I get her up from bed, in the morning, take her urine soaked Depends and gown off of her. Shower her and dress her. I put on her necklace and earrings. Then I take her to the kitchen and make her breakfast. I then fed her because she is unable to feed herself. I get the feeling that in my daily relationship with Nell that I have a stranger in my house. She doesn't know me, nor show any feelings, nor acknowledge any appreciation for all that I do. She is a stranger in my house. Or, I could say, I am a stranger in her house, and I wonder if she would want to ask me to leave if she could talk, but she can't. She might parrot a couple of words but that is all.

Last night I went to bed about 9:00 P.M. Nell had been in bed for two hours. She woke up when I got in bed. I changed the channel to Turner Classic Movies and the movie *Trip to Bountiful*. It was a beautiful message and an emotional movie. Nell really got into it. She showed herself to be so attentive. When the movie was over, I turned the TV off. Nell put her arm over me, like she used to do when she was healthy and whispered in my ear, "I love you." I was astonished to hear her give some words with compassion and showed a relationship. I did not feel like a stranger. I went to sleep with a new regard for my caregiving. I was wrestling with the idea of putting her in a nursing home, if all she is, is a stranger, and let someone else clean up her "messes," and feed her, and wipe her nose. And wipe her behind when needed. I thought a paid nurse could take care of this 'stranger." Then she turns over in bed and says, "I love you." I did not know that feeling was lurking back in her mind somewhere. Was it spontaneous and meaningful to me, her husband, or does she say that to others at E.A. Roberts? Does she feel an emotion and expresses it to a caregiver at E.A. Roberts as well as to the stranger in her home that takes care of her at that place? I guess I am a skeptic.

12/11/2016   Today is Sunday. Wynetta comes to our house on Sundays to stay with Nell while I attend worship services at Dauphin Way Baptist Church. I get her up and shower her, dress her and feed her breakfast. Then Wynetta comes and fixes her hair and puts her jewelry on her. She feeds her lunch and puts her on her bed for her nap, and I arrive home after worship and dinner about 1:30 PM, and Wynetta leaves. I let Nell sleep until about 3:00 P.M. I quit taking her to worship because It became too difficult. She didn't know what was going on, and so often, she would have an accident and I wouldn't know it until I would take her to the bathroom afterwards and put her in the Women's restroom, with her purse with Depends. It was a problem. I would ask one of the lady's to see that all went well. Some of the times they would tell me they had to clean her and put clean Depends on her. I knew that was difficult for them and for Nell. Because, I know when I clean her and put new Depends on her, she just stands and lets you clean her with no evident emotion. She offers no thanks, because she can't talk, or get any thought together to say it anyway. I just don't want to put her through this and other people either. I would rather they remember her as she was. Everyone loved her. She was so friendly and fun to be around. I did not want them to forget that Nell that they knew.

Nell has not shown any evidence of knowing me, or appreciate my feeding, bathing or dressing her. It is like taking care of a stranger. Would a man take a naked lady to the bathroom and take off her dirty Depends, sit her on the toilet, then shower and dress her. After that clean the toilet area, and feed her breakfast. Well, she is my wife of 62 years, so I do it. It is like doing this to a stranger, with no emotional connection except the memory of a life devoted to one another for all those years, so I do it.

12/16/2016   This morning about 6:30 A.M., I was reading in the living room when I heard a "thud!" coming from the bedroom. When I went into the bedroom, Nell was laying on the floor by her bedside, bleeding profusely from her head. I called daughter Carrie to come help me tend to her. Son-in-law Calvin came and we took her to the emergency room at Mobile Infirmary. They gave her a C-scan and put 13 staples to sew up the wound. Carrie and granddaughter Kim Coleman came to the hospital to see if they could help. We finally left about 10:30 A.M. with Nell who had a huge bandage around her head to keep pressure on the wound to hinder the bleeding.

Yesterday, I attended Nell's Murphy '53 class reunion Christmas luncheon. She was unable to attend. Thursday, the senior choir sang Christmas songs at E. A. Roberts, the Alzheimer Day Care facility. Afterwards, we all went to the Dew Drop Inn. Nell attended the choir presentation and I took Nell with me, and I fed her. She sat in a booth and we had a hard time getting her out of the booth. One of the ladies from the choir suggested to me not to subject her to going out in a restaurant anymore. We had a hard time getting her out of the booth, and feeding her.

We ran out of Donepezil medicine for Alzheimer's last night and I did not reorder, because, I do not think it is doing her any good. I have a hard time not giving it to her, but several Alzheimer's counselors suggested to me to discontinue it. Several nurses suggested I discontinue giving the regular dosage of blood pressure medicine. I can't do that at this time, but I have come to the place where I think I will discontinue the Donepezil. I will not refill the prescription.

(Note: Nell will go to be with Jesus one year from this date.)

12/17/2016   This is the third day not to give Nell Donepezil. Wednesday, 12/14 was the last day to give her the medicine. Friday morning, she tried to get up out of bed and fell and put a bad gash in her head. Today, she seemed to be as mentally alert as when she was taking the pill. But overall, we had a good day.

12/18/2016   When people call me to give me encouragement, they say, "It is like taking care of a child." They are comparing taking care of Nell with that of a child, in feeding, changing diapers, bathing etc. There is a difference. The child is taken care of with the hopes he or she will grow up and be a great contribution to the Kingdom, family and to society. But taking care of Nell who has Alzheimer's, is different, because there is no future hope for her, and therefore my hopes for her is not uphill but downhill in the body on this earth. My rewards and her hope are not in this earth, but in heaven. Ministering to her day by day, and really minute by minute is with the idea that ministering to her is like ministering to the Lord Himself, for Jesus said, when you minister to the least of these, you do it unto Him.

I took Nell out to the front porch about 9:00 A.M., this morning. She likes to sit out front and look at the cars go by and see the people. Not many of either, but she likes to sit out front. I generally let her sit out there for about 45 minutes. This morning after about 20 minutes, I checked to see how she was doing. For the first time, she got up and walked around to the front of the garage and was looking at the hanging flowers.

I was given a gift card to Zea's restaurant, so after church today, I went to Zea's all by myself. I didn't see any of the people I usually have lunch with from time to time, so I went by myself. I like to eat sometimes without the burden of feeding Nelda while I try to eat also. It is not relaxing to feed her and to wipe her nose, until she is through. So to not have to prepare the food and clean up after is a treat. But it is not enjoyable to eat by yourself. I am not going to do that again. If I cannot find someone to eat with, I will go home and eat with Wynetta and Nelda.

12/22/2016   Our daughter Kim came down from Huntsville on Tuesday and left this morning, (Thursday). She was 60 years of age yesterday. She came for her birthday and Christmas to be with Nell. I am not sure that Nell recognized her. She stared at Kim a lot as if somewhere in the past she recognized Kim, and tried to bring Kim to her remembrance. Kim left this morning to go back to Huntsville. I got Nell up to have breakfast with Kim and I about 5:30 A.M. We ate together and then went to the car as Kim left to tell her goodbye. I did not think she was in the departure of Kim with any emotion. Kim talked to me about some real things about Nell. What to do to prepare to take her to a nursing home when that time comes. She seemed to think that if I was ready to take her to a nursing home, she would be in agreement. She believed that Nell would be safer in a nursing home, as far as falling. She saw while she was here how diligent you had to be to watch her, because she would just get up and "wobble" before you could get to her. I know that Nell would be watched over, fed and bathed as good as I do (hopefully), but it is hard for me to be willing to take her to a nursing home. I feel like I would be giving up, and turning over the one I love to others rather than take care of her, at home. Although, when I take her to E.A. Roberts, she seems to get along very well. I think it would be the same in a nursing home. I think it would be harder on me than on her.

Her dad was put in Lynwood Nursing Home, and she never did like doing that. She did not like to go there to see him, even though she wanted to visit him. Even when I was the Homebound Minister at Dauphin Way Baptist, she would not go in to a nursing home with me because of her experience with her father. It was her desire, never to go to a nursing home for care.

It was a long time before she would accompany me to go in the nursing home to visit one of our church member friends. I don't think she would live long, if I took her to a nursing home. I think I would feel guilty for not taking care of her as I should and Nell trusts me to do the best for her in this life. Her life is in my hands.

People tell me that I have a life to live. I think about that and it comes to mind that Nell is my life.

We are going to go to Urgent Care this morning about 10:00 A.M. to take the 13 stitches out of Nell's head.

This is the first Christmas since Nell got Alzheimers that we have not been involved in the activities of Christmas. It is sad, because, in the past, Nell spent the whole year to get particular gifts for all the members of our family. This year I was just not "in it", to do that. Not only did I not have the spirit of the season, we do not have the finances to purchase any worthwhile gifts. Christmas is not Christmas – to me – without Nell's involvement. She doesn't even seem to care about the tree I have put up or the ornaments and manger scenes both in the house and outside. She is not in it, so I guess that is the reason I am not in it.

12/23/2016   I have a feeling I am being "closed" in with my caregiving. There are so many decisions that I need to make concerning Nell, and none of them are good. Because of her gash on her head due to her getting out of bed and falling, or maybe it was she fell out of bed and hit her head on something sharp. She may have hit the night stand or the bed rail. I can't let that happen again. I need to make a decision to get a hospital bed to put in our bedroom to keep Nell from another accident. Or, to put her in a nursing home, where they have beds with rails. I had Lisa Weaver from Kindred Care, make a requisition for a hospital bed. I am also filling out papers to have her take up a residence in a nursing home. I have already put application in for the "Little Sisters of the Poor," nursing home. They called and had an opening about six months ago, but I was not ready to move her. I am very hesitant to put her in a nursing home, anyway, because she said at one time not to put her in a nursing home.

But, due to the lack of help with Nell at times when I need help, the nursing home may be the only option. At times I feel overwhelmed, physically, emotionally and mentally, and need to get "away." My stomach is in knots, and I began to feel sorry for myself, and upset at others for not putting any priority in their lives for Nell's well-being (and mine). I know that family members have their families and jobs, so it is hard for them to see that "things" are not well in Nell's caregiving. They all think I am doing a good job taking care of Nell, so they have no real anxiety about the situation, as long as it looks good from a distance. I love Nell and want to do what is best for her. But, in her mind, I am just a stranger taking care of her. I am coming to the conclusion sometimes that being a stranger, any stranger can do what I am doing. However, Nell is not a stranger to me, so I want to do what is best for her, and my own mental well-being. If I put her in a nursing home, I would not feel good about it, then I would live with the guilt of putting her in a nursing home, and would feel worse than the oppression of the daily, minute by minute caregiving. So, this day, just before Christmas of 2016, I feel hemmed in with my caregiving responsibilities and decisions concerning Nell's well-being (and mine). It is easy for my friends and children to suggest what I need to do. I think if our children "took over" that decision and said "this is what we are going to do" I would be relieved. I don't think I would be so guilty. When we are all together on Christmas day, I am going to put the alternatives before them and let them come to a conclusion with me.

7:45 P.M. This morning after breakfast, it was nice outside. The sun was shining, so I took Nell to the front porch to sit in the sun. She sat there for about 30 minutes, while I cleaned the kitchen and swept up the floor in places. I checked on Nell several times to determine she was ok. Carrie came to our house to get a Christmas tablecloth. I went in the house to help her. It took about a minute, and when we came out front Nell was out of her chair. I ran around the corner and saw her laying on her back on the concrete driveway leading into the garage, bleeding from the back of her head. I put some cold rags on the bruise which was bleeding and took her to Mobile Infirmary ER. They took another CT Scan (which they did last Friday when she fell out of bed and cut her head badly on the top front portion of her head). This wound on the back did not need staples, but was described as contusions. They determined that her brain had no evident damage or bleeding. The nurse took out the staples from the previous wound and we went home arriving about 1:30 P.M. There did not seem to be any difference in her demeanor, maybe more subdued and sleepy. I just put her to bed, at 7:15 P.M. Hopefully, all will be well tonight, and she will rest well and be alert in the morning.

2017

1/2/2017   Nell has been doing better this last week, except some days Nell is sleepy all the time. Other days she is more alert and responsive to me in conversation. Friends visited one day, and Ray prompted her to respond to his request of her to remember and pray for Ray every day. In the past, he requested Nell to pray for her like that for a number of years. Today, he asked her, "who are you to pray for every day?" She responded, "Ray." I thought she did well, and it was unusual for her to comprehend what Ray was asking.

We went shopping today at Hobby Lobby, Bed and Beyond, and then had lunch at Morrison's. We had Black eyed peas for "Luck" for the New Year. Nell did very good, and when we got home, I changed her Depends and she layed down for a nap.

I have tried different women's diapers. The best one's are the Depends that I buy from Sam's. They will, mostly, hold her wetness during the night. If I use the Depends from Costco, I have to use a wrap around diaper over them. In the morning, Nell does not smell good, regardless the Depends I use, and I have to give her a shower first, before I dress her and give her breakfast.

I took Nell to the doctor this week to have him check her over, because she was groggy and sleepy since she hit her head several times this past week. There was a swelling on the area where she had the stitches. The doctor said it was a hematoma, and would go down. He said her sleepiness could be from the two big hits to the head in eight days, each time we did a CT scan for safety. He relieved my worry that the swelling might have been a seepage from inside her brain.

This is typed out as I have been going through a difficult time with the difficult place in our lives to figure out what is best for Nell's well-being. When I take my eyes off of her, she falls and injures herself. I am afraid she will break a leg or arm, or injure her head worse with the third hit on the head. My heart is broken in trying to make this decision so that it is not a decision that is self-centered. The decision is to put her in a nursing home, or continue as best I can. Or, to try to get more home care, or to take her more often to E. A. Roberts. God will lead, and things will develop to guide me in the way to go. I do have to get things ready for her to go to a nursing home, all the paper work and things like that. In case, first of all, if something happens to me, and second, if I am unable to continue the day to day care in home.

This was the first year we had Christmas at home, where we did not have a bunch of Christmas presents under the tree. Usually Nell gets all the presents and places them under the tree, and when the family members come to our house on Christmas, we give them their presents. This year we did not buy presents. We could not afford to buy presents for all the children, grandchildren and great grandchildren. They all have so much anyway, that we could not afford to buy any-thing worth anything anyway. Besides all that, I did not have the ability or energy to buy gifts. I told all my children, not to buy us anything, because there was nothing that was needed except prayer.

Nell had Alzheimers for about 18 months when I discovered this note in one of the dresser drawers, that I was cleaning out. It was written on a little note pad. I don't know when it was written.

I write this to you my dear husband for fear that a lot of my memory fails. Just so we can remember and pass on some of the treasures our life has [uncov-ered]. How were we to know, years ago on the corner where we met. That our lives would always be one. I do remember being so impressed, with the two stately handsome men in uniform. Not knowing on the Jan-uary 23 day when you and your friend Charlie, invited yourselves to my house. Even then – we weren't sure if the blonde was going to be my friend or Ruth's. Or who would have the privilege of the evening with the handsome young dark haired pilot. I am sure God was there and will tell us some day how his plan came together. How you spent an evening eating fruit cake that you didn't even like, "because you were hungry." Or, how it just happened that our 1st date was a mov-ie about Martin Luther. Or how you had to borrow $5.00 to get you back to your base which was only the beginning of several loans. Or how joking, later you used to tell your friends that you had to marry me to get out of debt. Or…how you have payed that debt to me with your unending love, compassion and under-standing.

You were always my families' favorite visitor, even from the very beginning. My mother loved cooking for you. Of course Daddy loved giving advice, even on how to fly, and at that time hadn't been in a plane.

Celie loved you, and her home was yours and that was a special gift that you shared with many of your cadet friends. With no car, many times we used Quitman's for our dates. I remember the night that you asked me to marry you. My youth was still a part of me, and I just thought it was a phrase that you passed on to a girl in every port. But that wasn't true, you did love me and the following months were very trying as we tried to communicate with you being transferred away to complete your training.

A very special time for me was when you asked me to come to Texas and pin your wings on, when you were commissioned as a 2nd Lt. in the U.S. Marines. I did feel out of place, younger than anyone else, mothers and wives were there performing this task, and then was me, a little 17 year old child, but one that truly loved you. The months that followed were eventful, planning marriage, saying goodbye to family and friends. During these months we had very little contact with any members of your family in California. But that was not important to me, because it was you I loved. I wonder how different our lives would have been on their part and mine if they had met me prior to marriage.

Do you remember the day we married? You just didn't understand why you couldn't be with me and see me. You never was familiar with tradition, and thought it was old wives tales. But when I walked down the aisle, it was worth it all to see the very large smile on your face. What a culture shock for the next few months. I did finally meet a brother in Cherry Point, who was a Marine Pilot also, who just about lost his composure when he saw me. Nothing like what you had dated through your college & high school years. This little skinny 94 pound southern girl, which he claimed it would never last.

This same little girl couldn't cook, never washed a load of wash and really wasn't good at making a bed. But, was willing to learn. I barely got over the cuts, bruises and tears of learning, when I found that we had another 1st on the way. What a year! Despite the culture shock of having to grow up now, that first baby was the very best. Six months after marriage you went to Puerto Rico. I was lonely with out you and overwhelmed by the event. You must have been too. Not many Pilots get grounded with morning sickness when I was pregnant. Then came that wonderful October morning when we had our son. I still remember what you were wearing when you walked into my room before dawn day. A red sweater- gray wool slacks, and grey & red plaid sox. You looked wonderful. From that point on I knew that this was the time to grow up and that I did.

There was the second child that was the perfection of our little family, before we left N. C. From that point on, only my deep love for you kept us together. There were about 4 or 5 years of where the Lord was dealing with you, and you were running from Him.

There was still another baby that bound us more closely together and you were such a wonderful father. There were monetary hard times that we did not handle well. But worse than anything were arguments on my Sunday Worship. But my love, God always wins. He touched your heart, and every thing was different. Thru it all we have had- big move to Alabama, from California. College for you. Move to Kentucky for seminary, and a new book could be written on Jeffersonville, and how it made this impression on our children. Move back to Mobile, and acceptance of Minister at CSBC. Doctor's program in New Orleans, and this without a move. Training and educating our children. Sticking together and supporting each other with all of the difficulties of pastoring a church for 22 years. You have received awards in college, awards after college, you have held many places in our community, city and our state that are impressive.

But I pray that the position that you have as my husband, father of Billy, Kim and Carrie, and grandfather to Brooke, Blake, Jonathan, Britanie, Kimberly, Stacey, Will, Mitchell, Laurel, and [Hannah's?] is the highest award that you can receive.

In our lives, you and I have many questions on "Why". My heart just cry's out within me, for answers, but some day – we will know. Until then, I just can't wait to look into the face of God and tell Him Thank you for giving you to me for my husband.

1/6/2017   I took Nell to the dermatologist on Wednesday to have several skin cancers removed. On Thursday, I took her to E.A. Roberts for the day. While there the head nurse, Laura Harrington, said Nell's bowels were compacted and she had to "help" Nell to have a bowel movement and there was blood involved in doing the procedure. I did not notice any more blood on the Depends, the next morning, so I believe she was alright. She was a little "draggy" the next day. On Friday, we went to Orchid Spa and had a pedicure, and then I took her to have her hair done.

1/9/2017   Last Thursday, the head nurse at E.A. Roberts, had to force Nell to pass a impacted toilet. Since that time she has not had a bowel movement. Tonight, Monday, I had to help her have a bowel movement by helping her. I only mention this for caregivers who may read this to help them in their care of a loved one. You can do this.

1/11/2017   I was told when drinking Ensure, she needed a daily laxative, which I started in the morning with orange juice. I had called the doctor and he sent a prescription for her to take once a day, to loosen up her bowels to where she could be more regular.

Nell has been sleeping soundly and when I try to get her up in the morning, it has been more difficult. Usually, when I tell her "time to get up," she repeats, "it's time to get up," and she gets up with my help. Now, she just continues to sleep. I have to do a lot of touching and turning and pulling on her to get her up, even though she has slept for twelve hours.

1/12/2017   I had an appointment with the dentist at 9:00 A.M. Then I took Nell to E.A. Roberts, while I attended an Alzheimer's lecture at their facility, around 10:00 A.M. Then we came home and had lunch. She did not respond very well to my relationship and conversation. She did not appear to recognize me. I laid her down for her nap, around 1:00 P.M. and got her up about 3:00 P.M.

We went for a walk after her nap. When we returned I gave her a snack, and a drink. She watched TV, most of the afternoon. I gave her a light evening meal, about 5:30 P.M., then laid her down for the night. I put a bandage on her nose with some medicine the doctor gave me for a cancer he removed on the bridge of her nose. I did not want the band aid pulling on her skin to make it uncomfortable, so I asked if the bandage was alright. She said her first words to me the whole day, and answered, "all right." I could not tell if she recognized me the entire day. She looked at me with squinting, staring eyes, that showed no recognition of me, in my estimation.

1/13/2017   I took Nell to E.A. Roberts today. When I picked her up about 4:30 P.M., Nurse Caitlin told me that Nell just wanted to sleep today. They tried to keep her awake, and asked me if she got enough sleep last night. I told the nurse that she slept 12 hours and mostly it was sleep. She did toss and turn several times, and place her leg outside the covers. Her leg was very cold, when I would try to put her leg back under the covers,

1/17/2017   Nell has been having trouble going to the bathroom. I gave her Miralax, in the afternoon every day since Saturday. I also give her a stool softener in the morning. It is the third day since she has had a bowel movement so I gave her a suppository. The first time I used it about a week ago, it seemed to help her, but since that day, I used it and to no avail. Maybe tomorrow, if no bowel movement, then I will try it again. A caregiver needs a nurses hat also. A nurse needs to know what is going on with your loved one.

The Homecare nurse told me that when an Alzheimer's patient has a problem with her bowel movement, that is evidence that the Alzheimer's has progressed to Hospice Care, for the patient. I have a meeting Thursday, Jan 19 with a Hospice Nurse to see what I need to be doing for Nell's well-being. The last week, she has been very difficult trying to wake her up in the morning after a night's sleep, or after a nap in the afternoon. Prior to this, several weeks ago, she was easy to get up in the morning and after a nap. Also, her sleep is so deep when I come to wake her in the morning. She will be laying on her side or on her back with her mouth open, and no evidence of breathing. I have been very upset to see her like that because,

I think, she may have died. I am afraid, I might go in to wake her up in the morning and she has gone to be with the Lord. Also, she is not able to walk as well the last week. She just verily shuffles. And she stumbles as we walk together. It is more difficult to get her in the car. I don't know what I would do, if she could not get her leg up and help herself get in and sit down on the seat. It is getting more difficult to feed her. She just will not open her mouth. She will keep her head turned away from me, and purses her lips closed and refuses to open her mouth so I am unable to feed her. She also, will not say words much, but when she does say something, it surprises me what she says, and understands. But that is very seldom. She used to parrot words, but seldom does that anymore.

The Beginning of The Loss of Speaking Words
1/18/2017 Last night after supper, Nell was sitting at the table moving a lot. I thought she was doing something in her Depends as was often the case when she performs those certain type of actions. Sure enough! I got her up and took her to the bathroom, and took her clothes off, all except her Depends and put her in the shower. She had the Depends "full." I did not like to clean up the mess, but I was glad she had a bowel movement, for it was three days, and I was worried, after giving her a mild laxative, a stool softener, and finally a suppository.

This morning, I got up about 5:00 A.M. and was reading the scripture and devotion, and it was brought to my attention about Job's experience, and He was calling into question God's reason for dealing with him the way He was doing. Last night I found out that two college students, I got very close to after graduation and over the last decade, lost their little daughter in an auto accident. I was devastated to know they are going through the loss of their sweet daughter in an accident. I thought, that in cases like this, and my case, we are left with the understanding, "The Lord gives, and the Lord takes away, blessed be the name of the Lord." That is hard to understand

and bear, but what is left? In a sense, I have lost the sweetest lady, that I could possibly have been blessed with some time ago. Once in a while, when I hold her when I get her up from bed in the morning, and at other times, I detect that she recognizes me with a little glimmer of a smile. Otherwise, most of the day, I take care of her, realizing that she does not know me.

I struggle at times whether I ought to take her to a nursing home where she could get better care, then I realize, that I am a unique person in her life. No one is quite like me as a caregiver to Nell. God is using me to bring Himself to her in a way that no one else can do. She brought God to me in a way that no one else could do as a young wife a half century ago, and so now it is up to me to bring God to her in many ways during the day: in cleaning up her messes, in dressing her, in feeding her, in walking her around the neighborhood, in taking her to E.A. Roberts, and picking her up, in giving her a shower, and washing her hair, in sleeping with her and cuddling with her at night like I used to. No. I am involved with her in many other ways, that no one can bring God to her in all these activities better than me. So, as long as God gives me strength (I believe He will) I will take care of Nell and minister God to her in my unique way. I will get her up from her night's rest in a few minutes, and will look in her eyes to see if she recognizes me. Sometimes she gives evidence that she does, and other times I don't believe she does.

1/19/2017   I woke Nell up this morning very easy, although she tossed back and forth all night long. She kept trying to get outside the covers even though it was very cool in our bedroom. I would feel her and she would be cold. So I would throw the covers back on her. She would just throw them off in a minute and lay on the covers. I did not like that because, she would wet outside her Depends and wet the covers, rather than on the pad provided for that reason. So, it was a battle to keep her on the pad, rather than on the covers.

1/20/2017 Kindred Care Home Hospice has just become Nell's Hospice care health group, to help bring home care help to me and Nell in her Alzheimer's disease. Deborah Palmer was the Representative to lead us in signing the contract.

1/21/2017 Nell has been very sleepy today, and very shaky on her feet. She did not eat well today. She didn't seem hungry, by pursing her lips and not wanting to eat what I prepared for her.

1/22/2017 This is Sunday morning. I got Nell up, showered her, washed her hair, put her robe on her and fed her breakfast. She has not had a bowel movement since Thursday, so I gave her a suppository. She had a slight hemorrhage. I put her in her chair in the bedroom to watch television, and went to the kitchen to put the breakfast dishes in the dish washer. I was gone about three minutes and when I returned, Nell was flat on her back beside the bed. I helped her get up and took her to the living room and sat her in her chair and raised the foot rest. She can't get out of this chair when the foot rest is raised. At least she has not got out yet.

Wynetta came about this time to care for Nell, while I went to worship at Dauphin Way Baptist Church. So she cleaned and dressed Nell.

People at church tell me that they are praying for me. I have been reflecting on their remarks that I am doing good as her caregiver. Others say that people are watching me to see how long I can continue caring for her. I wonder also, but I think, I am doing his because she is my wife of 62 years, and I married her for better and for worse. She needs me now, and I keep reminding myself that nobody can care for her like I can. I am unique in our relationship. There is no one who can relate to her, even though, mostly, she doesn't know me. I think when people see me faithfully caring for Nell as if it was completely a distasteful thing to care for her in all her needs, but, there are benefits to me also. I have her presence. She is company to me even though she does not know me most of the time. It is a blessing to me to hold her as I help her walk. It is a blessing to lay beside her in bed and feel her presence. She will put her arm over me, like she did in the past, and I feel Nell in those moments as if all was alright. I have great fear, to wake up and feel her during the night that she might have gone on to be with Jesus. She puts her arm out from the covers and her arm gets cold, or her foot is out and it gets cold, or when I come to wake her in the morning and she is laying on her side with her mouth open and doesn't seem to be breathing, I have a momentarily fear that she is gone. Then I touch her and see that she is breathing and moves. I have terrible feelings sometimes. I hesitate to speak it, but I have a hope that she has gone to be with Jesus. I feel guilty to have such a feeling, then when I notice she is alive, I thank God.

1/24/2017   I will tell Nell, "I love you," and she responds, "I love you." But recently, she just looks at me, and sometimes it is with a look, of "Who are you?" You can see it in her eyes. Last night when I got in bed, I remembered about the side rail that I did not put on her side of the bed to keep her from falling out of bed during the night. I tucked the covers in and around the side rail and leaned over and kissed her on her nose and forehead. I said "I love you." She just looked at me, but with no response. When I got in bed, I laid close to her and put my arm around her, and she tried to move near me, and kiss me on the cheek. I thought that was unusual. I think she could lean near me, and kiss me to show her acknowledgement of me, but she could not express her feeling verbally. She does not have the ability to express a thought. She could act out her affection, but could not speak it.

Today, Wynetta comes to be with Nell, while I attend the funeral of Kat Hanks, a very dear friend of ours. She was Von Ceil Turner's, Nell's aunt, friend and Sunday School teaching partner for many years at Dauphin Way Baptist. Kat and her husband were also in the same Supper Club Nell and I were part of for many years. There is one couple, along with Nell and I are the only members who remain. The wife of this couple is in a nursing home for therapy after she fell and hurt herself, and Nell has Alzheimer's. So the group that began a number of years ago with about 12 members is really down to two.

A lady in the neighborhood begins to clean our house today on a weekly basis. She is going to lightly clean, which includes cleaning the ceramic floors, vacuum, the carpets, make the bed and clean the master bedroom bathroom. We will see how that works out. I will clean all the other things that need cleaning, mostly in the kitchen, making the bed daily, and keeping things picked up. I thank the Lord for my family that helps to a degree financially, to be supportive in other ways, and is nearby when I need help with Nell. Mostly, Nell is under my constant caregiving presence. I can't let her out of my sight, nor allow her to walk without my holding her. It is getting harder now to feed her. She is very slow, and won't eat much. It takes so long for her to eat. When she doesn't want to eat a certain thing, she will purse her lips. If I wait a moment she might eat it, but if not, she is telling me, "I don't like that," or she is telling me, "I have had enough."

1/26/2017   Nell did not seem to be hungry today. I had several people from Kindred Care Hospice visit with us today. They would speak on sensitive subjects about Nursing Home, Advanced Directives, and other things about preparing for advanced funeral plans. I believe Nell could hear and comprehend most of what they were talking about, even though she could not have talked about any of the subjects.

I think the things that were talked about has caused Nell to be upset at me. She is upset and I think that what was talked about is the reason. I feel bad about it. I am getting ready to put her to bed. It is about 7:30 P.M. I think I will go to bed with her and touch her and tell her I love her. There is nothing sexually intimate involved, because that has been absent for several years. When she got Alzheimer's she, seemingly, had no desire, nor did I feel amorous as if I would be taking advantage of a partner that would be "used." I could not do that. So my affection is because I love her for who she is and has been for 62 years of marriage. There is nothing intimate in our relationship.

1/27/2017   Last night Nell kicked her feet to where it kept me awake. I tried to be comfortable. I asked if she hurt. I rubbed her stomach. Finally, I let her keep her body outside of the sheets. She was cold, but when I would pull the covers up, she would push them off. I pulled them down and let her be outside of the covers so she would not overflow from her Depends on the sheets on top. She was sleeping on a pad in case she does spill over, however, the pad absorbs it so I don't have to wash the sheets every day.

When I got her up she seemed to be angry with me. I think it was about the conversation I had the previous day with the Hospice nurse. I will need to be more careful. I showered her, dressed her, fed her and we went to E.A. Roberts about 10:30 A.M. I picked her up about 5:00 P.M. They told me that she had a bowel movement and it spilled over on her pants, which they changed before I took her home. When we got home I prepared one of the meals given to us by Meals on Wheels. She ate a couple of bites of green beans, a couple of bites of corn. She ate most of the hot dog without the bun. She just did not eat like she has been eating. E.A. Roberts told me she ate a good lunch so I did not worry that much.

I had a hard time getting her into the car when I went to E.A Roberts and putting her in the car when we returned home. It was difficult getting her in the car and getting her out of the car and into the house. It was difficult getting her to the dinner table. It was difficult getting her ready for bed. She needed to be cleaned after I brought her home from E.A. Roberts, so I gave her a shower. That was difficult. To get her dressed and into bed was very difficult. I am worried because it is getting harder and harder to move her around. Even getting a wheel chair will not take care of the moving her into and out of the car, and around the house and into the bed. I am fearful that I will have to make some kind of change in my caregiving procedures, if I am going to care for her at home.

1/28/2017   During the day, Nell was very tired, and sleepy. I had a hard time keeping her awake. I would try to walk her around the house. At one time I put her on the golf cart while I did some tree trimming. I had my back to her while I trimmed some limbs on the Confederate Rose, when I looked at the golf cart, she had fallen over onto the driver's seat, her head leaning on the arm rest. I don't know if she fell hard or easy, but she just looked at me in a helpless way, as I picked her up.

1/29/2017   This is Sunday, and it arrives with mixed feelings in my heart. I want to go to worship, but I feel guilty not taking Nell. But I know that she will have problems and it is a very difficult chore for me to take her. I think she gets more out of just looking at people. She doesn't recognize them, I don't think, nor does she get much out of the service, again, I don't think she does.

But, this is another day. I get up and feel depressed like every other day. My stomach is in knots, my mind is dark. I think only of Nell and how we are going to make it today. Today, I have Wynetta taking care of her until I get back from worship. My mind is on her and her needs. Should I enter her in a nursing home? I keep thinking that. But then I go on another day. I think I can care for her. I will try it a little longer. Then things happen during the day, and I come to a conclusion that I will have Hospice register her in a nursing home. But then at night as I lay there with her, I change my conclusion and decide to go on. Again, I am reminded that no one can care for her like I do. I realize at times that I am mostly thinking of myself, rather than her, and I get guilty about that. I think I would feel better about the caregiving situation if her children would come and take her shopping. Two of them are far away, and the other child is busy with work and her family. Nell has always been so self-giving, yet in these last days when she is lost in darkness, I would be blessed to see her children give her more attention, even the children living at some distance. But I know they have their problems being away from their work and family (Especially, the son's wife with multiple myloma and taking chemo). I am caught in a situation where I realize that this is the best we can get, and God meets our needs.

When I got Nell up, I got her ready for breakfast. I put new Depends on, her house coat and slippers and washed her hands. I used a liquid soap with a nice smell. I said "We need to get your hands to smell good." Nell said in response, "Smell good." It is unusual for her to speak at all. More important things I talk to her about, she will not say or respond in any way, but this time she did. Wynetta will give her a shower, wash her hair and dress her when she gets here at 10:00 A.M.

1/31/2017   Kindred Hospice aid and nurse came today to minister to Nelda. The nurse (David) brought Depends, wet pads, and a case of Boost. Her BP was normal. Pulse and O2 level was very good. The day was uneventful. We went for a walk in the morning and sat out front for an hour. I did have a difficult time getting her into bed tonight. She didn't try to help. She got half way in and just laid there. In trying to get her in she almost fell on the floor. I thought I was going to have to call Carrie and get some help. She got very afraid. I finally turned her in a manner where I got her head on the pillow. She laid in bed and was calm.

2/1/2017   Today, starts a new regime. Kindred Hospice sent an aid to our house to shower and dress Nell. They will do this on week days. Oh, that is such a help. It is not that I don't want to do those chores. I will still do them the days the aid does not come. But it is a relief not to have to do them every day, which I have done for several years. I have Wynetta coming at 10:00 A.M. this morning to be with Nell while I go to Senior Choir and lunch. Housekeeper, comes at 12:00 noon and cleans the floors and bathrooms. Once a month she will come now, and do a thorough cleaning, dusting, etc. This is so helpful. It makes it so Nell can stay at home rather than go to a nursing home. I have a nurse that comes to our home twice a week to take care of any physical needs that arise. He checks her BP and other measurements for her continued health.

2/2/2017   Yesterday, the housecleaner came the second time. She did not do a good job. I talked to her gently about the streaks on the ceramic floor, places under the breakfast table, the bathtub grime still in the bathtub. I will try several more weeks, and if she does not improve, I will have to discontinue her cleaning duty. I am feeling bad about it, because she had been out of church for some time and now she is going back to church and is so full of joy about it.

People ask me, "How is Nell doing? I am so faithless about her healing, knowing that it is said, that the disease of Alzheimer's is terminal. I feel like I need to tell them that she is going down gradually. I am faithless, in the matter, because I feel that is what people want to hear. I am faithless in the matter because, I want her to be with the Lord, in the manner in which she is living, I don't want her to be this way, and I want this disease to end. She is in darkness, and is just existing. She is like I am playing dolls with her. I shower her, I dress her, I feed her and sit her in her chair. I take her for a walk with her walker. But I am faithless in the matter, because I could be more insistent in praying for her healing, and believe that God might do a work of miracle and heal her. I do see some improvement, at times. Or, I should say, some light does come through at times. Why can't I be more faithful? Why can't I say in response to those who ask, "how she is doing"? to say, "She is getting better at times."

This morning as I got up about 4:30 A.M., I felt more exhilarated than I have in the past. I think it is because the aid is coming to shower and dress Nell. That is not a big problem, but for some reason, it evidently is a problem, because I feel relieved that someone else is doing it. I will continue to shower and dress her three days a week, (actually they began to shower her on the weekdays.) Wynetta will do it on Sundays. The nurse comes on Monday and Thursday of each week. That is a help to relieve my mind that all is going well with her physically.

I still have a hard time praying for her healing with all the information that tells me that Alzheimer's is terminal. I am torn between her going to be with the Lord, earlier, rather than later. I think some of my desire is selfish. I want to be faithful to do my best while Nell is alive. I want to do all I can for her, because there is no one else who has her interests more than me. She is entrusted in my care, and I am sure she trusts me to do my best, which I will.

Since this morning, Nell has not responded well. She is just staring and does not show any animation. I had a hard time getting her out of bed this morning, and a hard time getting her on the bed for a nap, and getting her out after her nap. I believe I am at the crossroads of making a decision to put her in a nursing home or having help at home. I cannot handle her physically by myself. She is hardly eating, and I add a Boost to her meal which is very slight. I am fearful what is going on in her. She can't tell me if she is feeling bad, or hurting anywhere. I don't think she is hurting or sick. I think the Alzheimer's is getting worse.

2/3/2017   We got up this morning, I showered Nell and made breakfast. She ate several bites of oatmeal, a couple of pieces of Conecah sausage. On the way to E. A. Roberts for Nell to stay, while I played golf, I gave her the drink Boost. When I picked her up she was very unsteady on her feet, difficult to get her in the car, and difficult to get her out when we got home. She seemed angry with me. When I fed her, she looked angry. She ate very little. So I gave her a drink of Boost. She drank it all. When I put her to bed, I tried a new way. I got a bed stool and had her stand on it so she could sit down on the edge of the bed, then I helped her lean into her pillow on her side. Then I rolled her over on her back. She sleeps all night on her back. It seemed to be easier and this worked out for her also. I kissed her on the forehead and told her I loved her. She just looked at me, with a searching look in her eyes. I asked: "Do you know who I am?" She still had that searching look, as if she was trying to remember. I said, "I am Bill, your husband who is a preacher. You remember me. I am the father, and you are the mother of three wonderful children. Do you remember me?" She just looked at me with a strange searching look, like who are you? Her look had a little fear in her eyes, like I was a stranger. I wonder if being at E.A. Roberts all day, she couldn't remember me, when I picked her up. I believe if I put her in a nursing home for a few days for respite for the caregiver, that when I picked her up, it would be a lot worse for her to recognize me, and I believe she would be more fearful of me. But, for my own health, when the time is right for me to take a few days to go somewhere, I will just chance the consequences, for my own well-being.

2/4/2017   Got Nell up, gave her a shower and sat her in front of the fireplace till breakfast was ready. I made a good sausage, and onion egg omelet. She ate most of it along with some grits. I took her to lunch about 1:30 P.M., to Foosakleys. She ate pretty good, but I had a difficult time getting her into and out of the car. When we got home about 2:00 P.M., I laid her down on the bed for a nap. She did not look as though she was "with" me at the restaurant. She just looked at the people. Every time I take her out to eat, I say to myself, it is the last time for her own dignity. I really don't mind it, but people stare, and act pitiful toward a person so helpless.

Overall, Nell had a good day. No accidents. We sat out front and had a cold tea and a half of an apple. Nell just stared at me with a strange look on her face for the longest time. Later in the afternoon, we watched a movie before supper. At about 7:00 P.M. I put her to bed. I devised a new way to put her to bed where her weight was not difficult to handle for me to put her in bed. I leaned over and kissed her on the cheek and told her I loved her. She looked at me and a slight smile came on her face.

2/6/2017   Sunday was a long day. Wynetta, Nell's Sunday caregiver did not show up. I did not successfully understand that she would not be able to attend Nell while I went to worship, so she did not come. But, other things were on my mind. Nell ate very little for breakfast. So I gave her one of the Boosts. She drank that, when I put her in her chair in front of the fireplace with TV. She always liked Chinese food, so we went to a Chinese restaurant and got a "takee outee" of food that I knew she liked. But when we got home and I tried to feed her, she only took about three bites. We ate supper at Carrie's and she only took several bites, and several bites of grandson Jonathan's birthday cake. During the night, she kicked her legs about every ten seconds, so I got up about 3:45 A.M. after about an hour of this disturbance. I checked her over and did not see any reason for her uneasiness.

My concern now is what do I do about her diet, for her to maintain physical health? The Kindred Care nurse is coming to meet with me today, to give me some directions. I don't want to put Nell in a nursing home if I can do what is needed here at home. I have been told, that when a person with Alzheimer's goes into a nursing home, they just go downhill fast. Later in the day Nell was feeling better. We went for a walk in the morning and in the afternoon. She does have matter in her eyes. The left eye is red. I put eye drops in the eye last night. No change today.

2/7/2017 I took Nell to E. A. Roberts and went to play golf today and got rained out after seven holes. I ate lunch on the way home. I came home and did some chores and it is now, about 3:30 P.M. I feel guilty not going and getting Nell from E.A. Roberts instead of waiting until 4:00 P.M. I could get her now, but they take good care of her, so I don't feel bad about her caregiving, just my being able to get her, and I rest for a while before I get her.

2/11/2017 Yesterday, Friday, Nell seemed quite alert, and spoke a few phrases, mostly parroting. Today, beginning with getting her up, it was a different situation. I could hardly get her up. She spoke no words today. I took her to J.C. Penney's to get her a valentine gift. We saw Karen, her understudy when Nell worked at Penny's in the personnel office. When Nell left, Karen took her place. Karen just made over Nell, but Nell just looked at her with no recognition. I tried to help her remember, to no avail. I took her down to Chick Fila for lunch. She ate a couple of pieces of chicken, and a couple of French Fries. I got her an ice cream cone. I had to feed it to her. She ate that from a spoon with no problem.

2/13/2017 It is difficult to get Nell to eat any of the food that is prepared for her. She will just eat two or three bites of food. I supplement her food with Boost. She will drink that. Sometimes I put ice cream with it. For breakfast I make oatmeal and fruit. She will eat that.

Kimberly Coleman, our granddaughter sent this message to Nannie by her cell phone to express her thoughts and feelings about her Nannie on Sunday night (2/12/2017) while we were at Carrie's house for supper. Even though Kim knew her Nannie could not comprehend the message, Kim wrote this, I believe, as an expression of her own needs

> Oh My Nannie, I never told you that day how pretty you were in that pale pink... Alzheimer's is one of the worst diseases. Nannie your mind goes to a place

where I can't imagine. You lose ability to hold a conversation at first and then all we can communicate to each other is echoed chatting. Now I sit here and talk to blank eyes, but I know inside is the sweetest soul. I went into JCPenneys yesterday and can remember the times we went to your office and I played with your switchboard looking phone, and your typewriter. I remember days we lived in your home and laid in your huge dining window in sunlight as you showed me where it was warm. I remember how much you loved cooking and Christmas. I miss so many things and can't bring my mind to stay there long or the pain overwhelms me. I think the hardest part is knowing my children will never truly know the best Nannie there ever was! I sat and watched my daughter play itsy bitsy spider on your neck and chest tonight, I hear her have her own conversations with you and even though you don't respond, she still can experience a few early childhood moments with you. She observes ever so closely as her patient Nana (Carrie)feeds you one small bite at a time, sipping tea from a straw slowly. You barely eat anything now. Nana sees Ryleigh watching you tonight and not comprehending why you don't speak. She tells you to say "Ryleigh". Some how, some where those letters mutter through your lips and the eyes of a child could light the room. I miss you so much. If you only knew how much your great grandchildren adore you too. I love you, Nannie.

When Nell and I were leaving Carrie's, Nell just looked at the children playing together. There was no change in her disposition, just a look that had no emotion or comment, but a disinterested look, yet a "needed" look of a great grandmother back in her brain somewhere. I was helping her walk and so I just stopped and let her look. Earlier in the evening, I was in the kitchen with Carrie and Kim, Nell was seated in the living room. We were talking in the kitchen, and I looked at Nell in the living room, and she was trying to get up from her easy chair, I am thinking, because she wanted to be in the conversation in the kitchen. So I went and brought her to the dining table so she could be near the kitchen conversation. Oh! How it hurts to see some response like that. She just sat at the table in a disconnected and in an unemotional manner, yet she seemed to want to be in the midst of things.

2/15/2017   The beginning of another day, Wednesday. This is one of the days the aid (Melissa) from Kindred Care comes to our house to bathe (shower) Nell and dress her. She does a good job and is nice and kind in her manner. She always fixes her hair so nice and when she is all dressed, she brings her out to present her to me, and I always make over her, on how nice she looks. I don't get any response from her. She is very stoic, but I think I detect a satisfaction that she looks nice, and compliments help her.

Last night when I was preparing to get Nell into bed, we went by the picture on the wall, that showed me kissing her when we got married. It was a picture that showed me in my Marine dress uniform, and Nell in a beautiful white wedding dress. I said to her: "Look at the picture there (as we both stood there looking at the picture) how beautiful you looked, in that wedding picture when we got married." I asked her: "Did you ever dream when you and I took the vows 'for better and for worse' that I would be taking care of you like this?" Nell looked at the picture and she had a very slight grin on her face, and her eyes took a life that she hadn't had for awhile. Then I took her to the picture of Billy, Kim and Carrie when they were preschool age and named the children to her. She looked with a slight grin, a look of pleasure and satisfaction came on her face. But she didn't linger, she was ready to get in bed. I helped her get in bed, and she laid down with her head on her pillow as I put the TV on a movie from TCM, that she watches till she goes to sleep.

2/16/2017   Wynetta is coming today to stay with Nell, while I go to senior choir at Dauphin Way Baptist Church. She is also going to do some cleaning as she can while being Nell's caregiver. Normally she comes at 10:00 A.M., but she is going to try coming a little earlier and start cleaning. She feeds Nell lunch and leaves when I return from choir and lunch, at 2:00 P.M.

Last night when I was getting Nell ready for bed, she had already had an accident in her Depends. So I had to give her a shower before I put her night clothes on. I was so patient with her, and I put her in bed in a loving way, so she would not feel bad about her "problem." Normally when I lay her down and kiss her on her forehead or cheek, I say, "I love you." She used to respond, "I love you." But she hasn't responded in that way for about three months. But last night when I expressed my love to her, she responded, "I love you." I was quite surprised, and of course pleased. She even tried to get close and with maybe an intimate "move" on me, in a very loving way. We have been celibate for over two years, so I was surprised. The reason I have been unable to be intimate with Nell is because in her mental condition, I thought it would be taking advantage of her in her inability to be involved.

This morning I fed her some cereal with strawberries and bananas with some yogurt. She ate most of that which I prepared. Melissa came and showered her, dressed her and did her hair really nice. I am playing golf in a minister's golf tournament today, so I will take Nell to E.A. Roberts about 10:30 A.M.

2/17/2017 Today is Saturday. Yesterday morning, Nell had these female symptoms. Dr. Ozwalt, urologist, said if she had problems on Monday take her to her obstetrician. Last night I forgot to put on the side rail on her side of the bed, and about 11:30 P.M., I heard her fall out of bed. I got up, turned the light on. She was laying on her stomach, and had pulled herself up on her elbows and looked up at me for help. I was able to pick her up and put her back in bed. I put up the side rail. She did not appear to be hurt in any way, this morning.

2/18/2017   Sunday. Yesterday was a good day for Nell. She is better than she has been in several months. She actually put a short sentence together. I took her to Café Del Rio for lunch yesterday. She walked in to the restaurant very good. She ate from my plate, and ate a good portion. However, last night she removed the covers and laid on them. The bed covers were all wet. I have had to wash all the bedclothes and her gown. I try to keep everything so clean and sweet smelling. I do not want it to smell like some nursing homes. Her female problem was in evidence last night but nor this morning.

2/19/2017   Monday morning. Nell had a good night, last night. I got up and I made pancakes, bacon, strawberries and grapes for breakfast. She ate most of the pancakes and bacon, a few strawberries and one grape. The Kindred Care Aid came to shower her about 8:06 A.M. I told her to watch for any evidence of her problem. If there was still evidence, then I would get a doctor's appointment to have this looked at. Everyone has said it was hormonal, but I am questioning that, and I want the doctor to take some samples and give me a proper scientific answer. The Aid (Melissa) from Kindred Care, said when she showered Nell, there was evidence of her problem. Nell got very white and almost fainted in the shower, she said. The Aid called the Nurse at Kindred Care, and she is coming to examine her, and if needed the nurse will call the doctor for an appointment and tell him what she has seen in her examination.

The office of Nell's obstetrician called and I set up a 2:00 P.M. appointment. She was examined, by the doctor, and was looked at with an ultra-sound, internally. They also took a blood sample to check her blood, to see if she was low on blood after this problem for 5 days. It was under his assumption that it was a hormonal problem. The doctor said it was partly, but mostly from a thin wall in her female area, possibly cancerous. He prescribed medicine to stop the bleeding, and medicine for hormones. Nell did very good in the exams and giving of blood. When we got home she would not eat but a couple of bites. I gave her a container of Boost, and put her to bed. She had evidence of her continuing problem in her Depends. I could not get the prescribed medicine, because it was too expensive, and the druggist tried to call the doctor and get a more reasonable medicine that I might give Nell. They will call in the morning. I hated not to buy the medicine. It was about $140.00, and another medicine is under $20.00. The doctor told me later just to use the hormone medicine that I have been giving her. I have been giving her this medicine for two days. I will give the third dose today. She had problems evident when I changed her Depends getting her ready for bed.

2/22/2017   This morning Nell did not have any evidence of a problem in her overnight Depends. She ate a small amount of oatmeal and banana this morning with about 3 small pieces of Coneceh sausage. The Hospice Aid is giving her a shower and dressing her, as I type at 08:30 on Wednesday.

I was reading along with my morning devotion, E.M. Bounds, complete works on Prayer. Each day I read a chapter. This morning the subject was on Prayer and trouble. There was a good verse noted:

> *O thou who driest the mourner's tear.*
> *How dark this world would be,*
> *If, when deceived and wounded here,*
> *We could not fly to thee?*
>
> *The friends, who in our sunshine live,*
> *When winter comes are flown,*

And he who has but tears to give,
Must weep those tears alone.

But thou wilt heal the broken heart,
Which, like the plants that throw
Their fragrance from the wounded part,
Breathes sweetness out of woe.

Isaiah the prophet says to the praying ones in trouble:

But now, thus saith the Lord that created thee, O Jacob,
and he that formed thee, O Israel, Fear not: for I have
redeemed thee, I have called thee by thy name, thou art
mine. When thou passest through the waters, I will be
with thee: and through the rivers, they'll not overflow
thee: when thou walkest through the fire, thou shalt not
be burned: neither shall the flame kindle upon thee. For
I am thy God, the Holy one of Israel, thy savior.

2/23/2017   When I got Nell up this morning and changed her Depends, it was the first time in a week, that she did not have any evidence of her problem. Thank God. The hormone she is taking seems to take care of the problem. Her blood pressure was a little high this morning. She just walked a little before it was taken, so that may explain the elevated pressure, according to Kindred Care Nurse.

2/25/2017   Yesterday, Nell stayed at E.A. Roberts, while I played golf at Magnolia Grove with several men from Dauphin Way Baptist Church. She ate some breakfast consisting of oatmeal, bananas and strawberries. I did not give her Boost, because I thought she ate enough of the cereal. When I picked her up from E.A. Roberts about 5:00 P.M., she seemed tired. The nurses said she had the same evident problem in her Depends, which I corroborated when I put her to bed later with fresh Depends. By the time she went to bed, she was very "drooped" over, and welcomed the bed at about 7:00 P.M. During the night, she would drape her leg and arm over me showing some affection, which she seldom shows in her waking hours. The only time I notice any connection with her, is at night when she seems to need some affection, comfort and security. She will put her hand in mine and I will hold it to let her know a mutual feeling of affection. I will also put my arm around her to let her know that I love her and it seems to give her comfort.

2/26/2017   Yesterday was very disconcerting. Nell was so weak, and not really being present. My granddaughter and a friend came for breakfast, and Nell just sat in her chair by the fireplace and looked at us eating, with little evidence of being emotionally involved. She is still in her problem. Not a lot, but evidence of it in her Depends and in the toilet after she empties her bladder.

3/2/2017   Thursday. The last several days Nell has been her regular self, with little unusual physical characteristics that is different than she has been the last several days. She is not eating more than a few bites of food I have prepared. Then I have to resort to Boost. She will usually drink all of the Boost. I gave her a boost for breakfast. She drank about a quarter of the amount. At lunch I mixed the balance with a scoop of vanilla ice cream. She drank a glass of the mixture, and I put her to bed for a nap. She is extremely tired and sleepy.

3/8/2017   This is Wednesday morning, and it is about 2:00 A.M. I could not sleep. I got up to make this comment for the last several days. For the last several days, there has been no change in Nell's normal physical well-being, mostly, the same. However, Monday night she showed evidence of her problem again, when I removed her Depends to get her ready for bed. During the night there was a little evidence in her

Depends when I changed her on Tuesday morning. At E.A. Roberts during the day, the nurse told me when I picked her up Tuesday evening that she had a little evidence of the ongoing problem during the day.

For the last month, Nell has cuddled with me during the night. When I say "cuddled," I mean she rolls over to my side of the bed and puts her arm around me and throws her leg over me. This is what she did before she showed any signs of Alzheimer's. Another thing, Tuesday, when I picked her up from E.A. Roberts, the attendants told me that Nell smiled at them several times during the day. When they said goodbye to her she looked at them and smiled.

Nell will not eat any solid food. This has been her habit now for several weeks. For the main I can get into her stomach, Boost and milkshakes. I gave her a cup of applesauce for breakfast Monday. She will eat some oatmeal at breakfast but not the complete amount in her bowl. I find myself buying groceries to try to meet her eating habits now. I bought ice cream bars and a two quart container of ice cream. I bought some fruit bowls and bananas, and strawberries to put in her oatmeal. She seems to eat the fruit along with the oatmeal. So I will try that for her breakfast.

3/13/2017 For the last several days, Nell has been constipated and this morning after some time on the toilet she was able to have some relief. She looked so hurt and pitiful, unable to talk, but I could see her anguish on her face. She will not eat anything. I gave her a bottle of Ensure for breakfast. For lunch I mixed it with Activia and ice cubes and mixed it in a milkshake. She was weighed by the Hospice Aid this morning. She weighed 133.2 lbs. I took her for a walk around the cul de sac this morning. She was "winded" when we got back to her chair. The nurse from Kindred Hospice came to visit about 3:00 P.M. David, our regular nurse could not come and the substitute nurse came. It surprised me when the nurse, who w was the substitute, came. She grew up in the Cypress Shores Baptist Church where I was pastor. I knew her as a little girl; I knew her parents and brother. I was so glad she came and treated Nell. She did it with so much affection. Maybe she will take David's place, although David was a good and kind and helpful nurse also.

EATING MAINLY LIQUIDS

3/14/2017   It is 3:30 A.M. Tuesday. I went to bed around 9:00 P.M. last night and slept till about 3:00 P.M. I have a troubled spirit about feeding Nell. She will not take a bite of most any kind of food. It is all drinking. She has lost weight and I have tried to use some ingenuity to put calories in her Boost and Ensure to keep her weight up. When Ashley came, she told me that soon she will not even want to drink through a straw, or from a cup. I am taking Nell to a local nursing home for five days of respite for me while I go to the gulf. I have misgivings about doing this. But, I am so committed in other ways, that I will go through with this. I am afraid, that she will stop eating while I am absent for those five days. They are not able to keep their eyes on her, like I do, and she might fall and break her leg. Also, she might not have any knowledge of who I am when I return to get her. Our relationship might be entirely different when I pick her up. She may have deteriorated so much that she will be more difficult to care for at home, and I will have to take her back to the nursing home for good.

3/15/2017   Wynetta did not come for her Wednesday appointment, so I am going to take Nell to EA Roberts, while I can attend the Senior Choir rehearsal at Dauphin Way Baptist Church, dinner following. Laura Herrington of EA Roberts called yesterday to talk about her obstetrician's medical diagnosis of Nell for the problem she was experiencing. I told her that he prescribed a medicine for hormones and saw a possibility of cancer through a ultra sound. He did not want to take a biopsy, because he said that more than likely you would not want Nell to go through the surgery if needed, along with Chemo, or radiation at this stage of her Alzheimer's disease.

3/16/2017   Thursday morning, 4:10 A.M., and I have been up since 1:45 A.M. Nell continued to throw her arm and legs over me. And as she was next to me I remembered what the nurse told me several days ago, that while now she was only drinking Ensure or Boost or water, or milk shakes through a straw, and not eating any solid food, there will be a time in the future when she will not even drink through the straw. I began thinking about the "directive" that she signed before she lost any ability to think right. Well, now I am faced with the decision to continue giving her calories through her vein or not getting water or Ensure or anything in her, and let her die from starvation and thirst. Should I continue to take care of her at home during this period, or should she go to the hospital. I don't know what the procedure will be to help her through this stage until she passes to the Lord in Paradise. She can't talk and tell of pain or hurt, so this is a hurt on my part also, though assuredly, not like her pain. (As I am editing this, I add here that my worry was her imminent death, but she did not die until December 17.)

3/18/2017   Yesterday (Friday) afternoon, when I changed Nell's Depends, she had evidence again of this reoccurring problem in the Depends. I put on fresh Depends when she went to bed, and this morning there was no evidence of her problem. But, all day yesterday, she was very sleepy. She was difficult to get up from bed in the morning. She wanted to sleep right after breakfast. When I would put her in her chair to watch TV, normally she would watch the show, but yesterday, she just went to sleep. She slept 12 hours last night. Today, she seems quite alert. But she is really down, from what she was last month or weeks ago. She has no energy. She can't hardly keep her balance when I walk her. She won't eat anything except Ensure or Boost. She will drink water through a straw. That's it.

3/20/2017   When I wake Nell in the morning, I try to be cheerful. That is tough when you see her sleeping, and when I awaken her, she screws up her face. She does not smell pleasant. And it is difficult to get her up from the bed and her feet on the floor. She helps me all she can, but she is still dead weight. I bring her to my chest and cheerfully say to her, "This is the day the Lord has made, rejoice and be glad in it." It is 6:00 A.M. and a Monday. This is the Monday I am taking her to a nursing home for a week. Kindred Care has made those arrangements, and I am going to the gulf for 5 days on "respite" leave. I don't know how this is going to work out. I have some fear that Nell will go down rapidly while I am gone. We Will See.

3/21/2017   This is Tuesday. Yesterday, I took Nell to the Nursing Home Residence for five days of respite care for me. I left her there in a chair sitting beside her bed. Only a television, and it was off. She looked so pitiful as I left. It was hard to leave her. Now Tuesday morning, I wonder how things went with her all day yesterday, through the night, and now morning when I usually get her up. I am just expressing my feelings this morning. Did not sleep well last night. What does she feel? Was she hurting when I left. Does she know where she is? Will she recognize me when I return? Oh, this is a tough time in our lives, and I don't know that what I am doing makes it more difficult or better in the long run? I hope I am a better caregiver after this week "off."

3/22/2017   I have been to the Gulf for two days. I talked to Calvin and Carrie, who have been to see Nell at the Nursing Home, and both times she has been in her night clothes in bed. I don't think they have dressed her, and walked her. I called the nurse at the nursing home around 9:00 A.M. on Wednesday morning (today), and she said all was well with Nell. I asked her to make sure they were walking her in the morning and afternoon. She said they would do that. I say that hopefully they will.

3/24/2017   I will be picking up Nell today at the Spring-hill Nursing Home. It will be interesting to see how she is after five days in a memory care unit. This morning (Friday), I don't have any misgivings about being absent from her these five days. I hope I don't have any after I pick her up and see some drastic change. It has passed through my mind after being gone from Nell's presence, these few days, that the absence (if it comes to that) when she passes from this earthly existence, it will be similar. Now, I know that I will pick her up today at the Nursing Home, but when she goes to be with the Lord, I will not be able to go and pick her up and be physically present with her. I am getting a little preview of what it is like to be absent from her, but knowing that I will be with her today will be a great comfort and joy to me. I don't know if there will be any comfort and joy with her in her mental condition. It would be great to me, if I could see something in her expression or in her eyes to show me that she is glad to see me. I think it will be a hurt to me, if there is no recognition or expression of some sort after being absent from each other for these five days. Especially after being with each other 24 hours a day in close relations in everything. I believe I will be able to absorb the hurt after taking care of her in the past days with seemingly no recognition.

3/24/2013   I brought Nell home today. She was laying in bed asleep, at the nursing home when I went into her room about 2:00 PM. I woke her and walked her to the car. She went back to sleep in the car. When I got her home, I took her to the bathroom and changed her Depends. I brought her to her chair in the living room. I sat her down, gave her a sip of water, and she went to sleep. I have tried to wake her several times the last several hours. She opened her left eye once, and then went back to sleep. Her eyes do not look good. Her eyelids are drooping and can barely get her eyes open. There doesn't seem to be "life" in her eyes. A great emotion of desperation came over me that she may never open her eyes again. Unless she was greatly tired, I don't know why she won't wake up unless she has been drugged. I will try to feed her some Boost in an hour (5 :00 PM) and see if she will sip some of the energy drink. I do believe that she is in her last days, maybe hours. The Kindred Care nurse came about 5:00 PM, and took Nell's vital signs and they were all good. Nell opened her eyes and actually smiled at Candy, the nurse.

3/25/2017   The next day after being at the nursing home for five days, Nell was still drugged. When I got her up from bed, she was difficult to wake her. She was very shakey and unstable to shower. But I thought it would help wake her. She smelled, as if they did not use underarm deodorant.

It was not until about 2:00 PM, the next day that Nell came around to be somewhat alert. I got her up from her nap. She could hardly walk. I had to – practically – carry her to the living room. I will have to get a chair in the bedroom to let her sit in there with her feet up, rather than try to walk her to the living room, until I see that she is strong enough, if ever she will be. I sat and looked her in the eyes today, and thought to myself she was really sick and would not live long. I asked if she understood that she was really sick to squeeze my hand and she did grip my hand to acknowledge what I said. Then I talked to her about our past, our marriage and children and events in the past. I think she understood, even though she is unable to talk. There was no emotion in her eyes and that led me to believe she may not have understood. There is no way to tell if she knows what is going on or does not understand.

3/29/2017   Wednesday. Nell has been more alert and strengthened since leaving the nursing home. Yesterday she spent the day at E.A. Roberts. The nurse told me that she had a red spot on her rear, like she had been sitting down on a hard surface. They put medicine on the spot. It was difficult for me to get a can of Strawberry Ensure down last night. When I gave her a pill and a drink of water, she did not swallow it, She later (a minute) spit it out on the bathroom floor. She slept well last night and tended to cuddle with me during the night. She would throw her leg and arm over me. At times she would grab my arm and pull it over her.

3/30/2017   Nell was evaluated by the Kindred Care Hospice nurse today, and was found to be in good physical condition, except she has not been to the bathroom for four days. I gave her Miralax in the morning with a stool softener, and today, I will give her some more Miralax in the mid-afternoon. Kim, the nurse, said if she does not go to the toilet by Monday, we will need to do something else. So, I will do what I can this weekend to see that she goes to the bathroom.. She seemed to want to sleep everytime I sat her down and left her quiet, even if she was watching a movie. She smiled a big smile to Kim her daughter from Huntsville, when she arrived. I think she remembered her kind spirit.

4/10/2017   All seemed to go well today. Nell wanted to sleep more than usual. She also, was a little slow in sipping her Ensure. She was also a little more wobbly and weak in walking. I can tell that daily there is a little slipping in a lot of ways. I am going to go to the Lighthouse for dinner tonight with Nell's 1953 Murphey class alumni. She is staying with a neighbor lady at her house, then Carrie will relieve her.

4/11/2017   We went shopping today. Nell stayed in the car while I went in to the various stores and purchased an item or two then came right back out. I brought a can of ensure with us for her lunch and I purchased a pizza at Mellow Mushroom. I parked at Springhill College in the shade and fed her while I ate a portion of a small pizza. Then we came home and tried to get Nell on the bed for a nap. Usually she steps on a raised step and lays down on the bed. But today as she tried to step up on the step, her legs collapsed and she went down on her knees. I gripped her under her arms and we tried it again. I was able to get her up on the bed. After her nap we went for a little walk on the street with her walker. She got so weak, I didn't know if I could get her back into the house on her chair. Soon, I will not be able to take her for a walk. Nell is getting weaker, no matter what I do. Her whole life is getting weaker, her eating, walking. It is day by day. Soon she will be bedridden, and I will not be able to shower her. I know this sounds pessimistic.

4/12/2017　　Took Nell to E.A. Roberts today, while I went to Senior Choir and had lunch with several choir members. I did some shopping and then picked Nell up approximately 2:30 P.M. She seemed alright when I drove her home. I put her on the bed about 3:00 P.M. and she slept until about 4:30 P.M. When I got her up we took a short walk. She was breathing so hard, that I shortened the walk to about 30 yards. I sat her down on the front porch and got her some cold water to drink. She drank her Ensure for supper along with several spoonsful of icecream. I put her to bed about 7:30 P.M. to watch a movie on TV until she goes to sleep. However she finally went to the bathroom this morning before I showered her. I changed her when I brought her home from E.A Roberts, and then again when I put her to bed. In the morning, the Nurse Kim will be here, about 9:00 A.M. I will attend the lecture at E. A. Roberts at 10:00 A.M. in the morning. The subject is: The Stresses of the Caregiver. Nell will stay at E.A. Roberts.

4/13/2017　　Got up early and ate breakfast. Kim the nurse came and gave Nell a physical checkup. She was normal in the sense, there was no change from yesterday. We went to the lecture at E. A. Roberts and returned to have lunch. Afterwards, Nell took a nap. She sat out in back on the patio for about an hour and I bought her back into the house fo her nap. She watched TV after her nap. She ate some ice cream with a half of a banana, and a can of Ensure for supper. Tomorrow I will take her to E. A. Roberts while I play golf at Springhill Golf course. Then later in the evening will attend the Good Friday Services at Dauphin Way Baptist. A neighbor lady will sit with Nell while I attend the services.

4/14/2017   Nell stayed at E.A.Roberts today, while I played golf at Springhill College Golf Course. I had a toothache through the night and almost did not go to play golf. God healed the pain at the time I needed to make a decision. I got up this morning after tossing and turning through the night with a toothache. I asked Carrie by a text message before I went to bed if it was alright to take an Ibrupofen for a toothache. She said yes, but it didn't seem to help. I got up in the morning about 4:00 AM, with the tooth aching and I considered cancelling playing golf with a foursome at Springhill Golf Course today. Carrie left a message on my I phone that I could call our dentist, and even though their office is closed today (Friday), leave a message and he will send a prescription for an antibiotic. That is my intention.

I went into the kitchen to get me coffee to drink while I did my morning devotions and prayer. While I was pouring my coffee, I prayed as if God was near me in the kitchen - He was - and I prayed casually for Him to heal my toothache - or to take away the pain - not sure, what I asked. But, when I sat down and began reading my devotion I felt a wave of warmth feeling flowing down the side of my head and my cheek where the ache seemed to be, and I got sudden relief.

I decided to go ahead with my golf plans. I will get Nell ready and take her to E. A. Roberts and go play golf. I believe God has a reason to heal or to bring relief from the toothache beyond my own displeasure. It remains to be revealed, but it will be a joy to find out and to be a part of what God is doing today in which I can be involved. Now, I am not being faithless to phone my dentist to send a prescription of an antibiotic to the drug store. I will continue to pursue the tooth infection remedy, and if God has healed the infection, I will be thankful. If it is His will just to take away the pain while I continue my regular plans, I will be grateful for that. If the pain reoccurs after what God has planned for me today, I will take the antibiotic to combat the infection, if still there, and thank God that I have an antibiotic.

I called my dentist and he sent an antibiotic and pain medicine to Walgreens. I started on the medicine about 3:00 P.M. I am now getting ready to go to the Good Friday Services at Dauphin Way Baptist.

4/15/2017   We got up around 8:00 AM this morning, showered, washed Nell's hair, dressed her and sat on the patio. I fed Nell an Ensure. She drank a half of can, and I continued to feed her through the morning until she drank the whole can. I opened another can of Ensure about 11:30 and she drank about a third of a can. I gave her some ice cream and some fruit cocktail. She ate about six bites and refused to eat more. I tried to get her to drink water. I changed her Depends about 3:15 PM. Her Depends were not very wet since I put her Depends on her this morning. She has been sleeping in between our activities; sitting on the back patio, watching TV, and eating. I can judge that her life force is deteriorating. It is 4:15 PM, and we have not left the house all day.

I still have a bad toothache. There was a period about 11:00 AM where I thought I would cook steak on the grill for my meal tonight. Then my tooth became worse, and I can't put any pressure on it. I took another pain pill. But I will cook the steak and put it into the freezer and eat it later. I am in pain and sleepy.

4/16/2017   Easter of 2017. Got up and dressed half way, then got Nell up, showered her and dressed her. Then I dressed mostly, and took Nell into the Kitchen to eat at seven in the morning. It is seven o'clock in the evening, and we returned from granddaughter Laurel's house where we had supper. Brought her home and cleaned her. Her feminine problem reoccurred earlier this afternoon, so I had to give her a shower, and get her ready for bed. I remembered I did not feed her the evening Ensure. I will have to do that before I lay down to sleep.

4/17/2017   Monday morning. I did feed her a can of

Ensure while she was in bed last night about 8:00 PM. This morning she went to the toilet. When I tried to feed her this morning, she was resistant to drinking the orange juice and the Ensure. She didn't take all of her blood pressure medicine, that she takes with the juice. I tried to put the pill in her mouth but she would not open her mouth. She finally drank the juice and her Ensure with her medicine . Melissa came and is giving her a bath. The nurse Kim should be here soon.

4/18/2017 Yesterday, I spent my day taking care of a molar on the lower left side of my teeth with an endodontist. Nell went with me to the dentist and waited in the doctor's office on a couch. Most of the day, Nell would not drink the Ensure that I brought along with me to feed her. She is slowly resisting my feeding her the Ensure that I try to get her to eat. Little by little it is getting harder for her to drink the Ensure. I am getting nervous about her inability to swallow. She takes a sip at a time, therefore it takes about an hour to feed her. Or she may quit sipping after she drinks about a half of a can of Ensure. This morning I was able to get her to drink her orange juice and take her pills. She also drank most of her Ensure. It took from about 7:17 A.M. until 8:00 A.M. to finish her breakfast.

4/19/2017 Nell has not done well this Wednesday. No energy. Even though she ate her Ensure for breakfast and lunch. But mostly she has been sleeping. We did take a walk, and I let her sit out front on the patio while I mowed the grass in the front, and sat her near the back door while I mowed in the back. She slept mostly even with the TV on. She got up this morning with her feminine problem. I have been giving her the pills at night for her hormonal need according to her obstetrician. It mostly helps but then about every ten days, it will reoccur for about two days. The medicine stops the problem, mainly.

I changed her Depends about 11:30 A.M. after she drank her Ensure. She needed to be cleaned and showered. She had an accident going to the toilet. I had to wash the throw down rugs, and mop the floor after I bathed her and got her redressed. She is now taking a nap.

The job of the Caregiver never ends. I have to get her Ensure and feed her lunch, which takes about an hour, sip at a time. Washed, dried and fold the colored clothes and put them up. When you are the caregiver for an Alzheimer's patient, you are occupied most of the 24 hours in the day. Some moments are casual, and other moments are intense. The caregiver has to take opportunities during the day when other duties can be taken care of.

4/20/2017 This is Thursday. It has been a terrible emotional day as the caregiver for Nell. My plan was to take Nell to E.A. Roberts while I played golf with the Minister's golf tournament at Heron Lakes Country Club. I then was to pick her up after the golf tournament and take her to her obstetrician for an ultra sound because Nell has experienced her feminine problem for at least four days. Kindred Care thought she should be looked at to determine if the hormones her obststrician had recommended she take each day from back in February was to be continued in lieu of her continued problem every ten days or so, and it would last for several days. Now it has lengthened into four days. E. A. Roberts phoned me to come get Nell about 11:30 A.M. They said she had a runny nose and her left eye had liquid running from it. They did not mention she was experiencing her problem, though she was. So I left the golf game about through nine holes. I picked Nell up and her obstetrician's office said I could bring her right in. We went in about 1:15 P.M. After about an hour, her obstetrician took me aside and said for me not to give the hormone tablet to her anymore and he believed she would be alright. I was at my emotional stress point because she could not walk into his office. She could hardly open her eyes, and looked listless. I started to ask her obstetrician to put her in the hospital because I did not believe I could continue to care for her in her condition, listless, eyes watering, nose running, feminine problems, and I choked up in the doctor's presence. He tried to console me and offer encouraging words, and told me not to put her in the hospital and to take care of her in the home with the help of Kindred Hospice nurses. I brought her home and took her to the toilet. When I took her Depends off, her problem was awful. I took her to the shower and cleaned her, I finally had to put her Depends on in the shower room. I put another Depends on over the Depends. Then I dried her legs and put her night gown on and got her ready for bed. I put her in the bedroom chair with the legs up. I had to put the rugs back in the washer and redo them when I had washed them again. I sat her down in her chair and raised her legs up, and turned the TV on to a movie. She just looked at me with endearing and tired eyes, as if she was saying, "Thank you for taking care of me." Or maybe she was saying, "Pray that the Lord would take me." It was a very emotional episode, and a day that was emotionally depressing, and hurtful to see her like that.

4/21/2017   When I changed Nell's Depends at noon, after her lunch and before her nap. She had feminine issues. She also had an accident. I showered her and put on new Depends, and laid her down for her nap. I called her obstetrician and his nurse called a prescription to Walgreen's to stop the feminine problem. The nurse from Kindred Hospice, Kim, came and took her vital signs which were normal. I am giving her Claritin for her allergy problem.

4/22/2017   This is Saturday. I took Nell to Hobby Lobby about 11:00 A.M. today. She always liked to shop, so I got a wheel chair and took her in and rolled her up and down the aisles. She seemed to look at things. I want to make her life normal, even though I know that it is not. Maybe it is more for me to be in a normal relationship with Nell. I do not want our relationship to be more of a hospital type. Like, I am taking care of physical needs all the time. But, this morning when I got her up she looked more listless than usual. After a while, she seemed to perk up, but later, her eyes gave her away as being very tired, and close to death look. It has made me quite emotional today. Things I saw on TV, would choke me up so easily.

There is a basket on the wheel chair and when I raised it to get Nell out of the chair it fell and hit Nell on the head and caused a small wound. It bled and caused me and the employee at Hobby Lobby some alarm. We put a small bandage on it to stop the bleeding. It was pitiful. I was careless to not see that the basket could fall and she looked so hurt at me for allowing that to happen.

I began to make plans to speak to our children to come and spend a day a month with Nell. I would tell them to sit down on the couch with her and just hug her and talk to her eyes. Then hug her for an hour or so. The reason I think that would do the kids good, and Nell good because it does good for Nell and I when we go to bed at night. When I get in bed and hug her and tell her I love her, during the night she will roll over against me and throw her arm around me in affection. The only time during the 24 hours of all the caregiving, that she shows any human feeling is at those times at night. That is a good reason not to take her to a Nursing Home, if I can avoid it.

In the morning I will get up about two hours before I go to get her up. She is oblivious to it. It is about 7:00 A.M., she looks like she is dead. When I look at her, I almost wish the Lord was gracious to take her, then I am ashamed for thinking like that. I wonder sometimes if I want her to continue on living because of wanting to keep her alive for myself. No, for herself, for what reason? I ask myself. She suffers during the day. Not in pain, that I know of, but her eyes show no joy, only being here. I clean her, even when she is having her feminine problem. When I shower her, and clean her because of her feminine issues, she is oblivious to it. I get her dressed and sit her down to watch TV during the day. I feed her during the day. She is oblivious to what is going on, but she is HERE. I think – do I want to help her to live, because I would be lonely without her, even as I am taking care of her as a little baby, but with no response. I think I am selfish to want to make her live longer, because I would miss her company, even though there is no responsive relationship. But, when she is in her chair, watching TV, or sleeping on the couch for her nap, she is there. When she is gone, there will be no one there. She will be in heaven, and I will be in this house, looking at a vacant chair, or couch or bed. No one in bed, to throw their arm around me, to feel, and to show, maybe, a sense of appreciation and care on her part for all I do to make her last days comfortable. Oh, how selfish I am. When I look at her droopy eyes I get emotional and start to choke up in tears, because I know it won't be long.

I wish all the children and grown grandchildren who knew Nanny when she was so vibrant, and all she thought about was-them, that they could experience that person again. She always shopped for their Christmas presents all year long. She would see something and say, "I need to get that for Rachel." I would say, "You already got Rachel a gift." She would say, "But Rachel needs that." When I think about that, repeated so many times with the other children and grand and great grandchildren, it makes me choke up. She was so thoughtful. She needed nothing. She never went to a beauty salon, or had her nails done, until I took her when she had Alzheimer's. She took care of herself, and me when it came to grooming. I don't believe I ever went to a barber when I had hair, after we were married. Never went to a pedicurist for my toes. Nell would clip my toes and sometimes to the quick. I would bleed for days. But I never went to a pedicurist until Nell could not do my toenails. That was after she got Alzheimer's.

She loved our new home, but soon after we moved in she began showing signs of Alzheimer's disease. Some blame the move from our home in Cypress Shores, on the rapid movement of Alzheimer's. We lived in the other house for some 40 years in Cypress Shores. The shock in the emotion of a woman moving may trigger some fear and insecurity in their brain. But, my point is, she has not enjoyed her new home in an awareness of it, like she should have. Maybe she was conscious of her new home in Saraland, for two years, then I believe it began to fade. I began to take care of her. She became incontinent in the first stage of Alzheimer's then I had to move her into Depends. That was a problem also. When I think about all of this, it chokes me up. She deserved better. She was always so self-giving. Holiday dinners and family get-togethers were always planned and cooked by her and served in our home in Cypress Shores. At the last, even before we moved, It was getting difficult for her to do it all. The children began to help more and more. Today, has been an emotional day for me, because, I think, Nell does not look good today.

4/23/2017   Sunday. I went to worship today, and Andrea was the Caregiver. After worship I went to lunch with Billy, my son at Dreamland in Mobile. After lunch he visited with Nannie and Carrie and I in the afternoon. All went well with the caregiver and Nell. Nell seemed to pay attention to being with the family. I changed her Depends about 2:30 P.M. and there was evidence of some feminine issues again.

Tonight when I put Nell to bed, it was an emotional thing. I got her all ready and took her to the toilet. Then I put on her Depends and brushed her teeth. I gave her a Claritin pill and water to wash it down. As I started to dry her mouth, she spit up all the water she had in her mouth. I looked for evidence to see if the pill came out, but no, she seemed to have swallowed the pill. When I dried her mouth, she looked at me with endearing eyes, as if to say, "I didn't mean to do that, thanks for not scolding me." I led her to bed, and laid her down. I tucked the covers around her, and she looked at me with alert eyes and a thank you smile. Not a real smile, but a countenance smile, not a frown. It was a very slight smile. A smile that I could verily make out, but it wasn't the usual look of distrust, or hostility, even. But the emotion of it was in my thought as I had finished cleaning her. When the Bible says, two shall become one, I am that functional part of you now. I am the part that keeps you clean. We are one in that. Our visits to the toilet are as one. What oneness! Tomorrow begins another day. Twenty four hours of oneness.

4/24/2017   This morning Kim, Kindred Hospice nurse and I was talking about some of the things that I mentioned above concerning Nell's possible death, and my feelings about this event. We just got back from Orchid Spa where she got a pedicure and manicure and color red added to both the nails on her hands and toes.

4/25/2017   Tuesday. Nell looked a little better today, although she will go to sleep easily. I sat her out front in the patio this morning to finish her Ensure. She sat there for about an hour while I did some light yard work around the patio and back fence. Then I brought her in to watch a movie about 10:30 A.M.

4/29/2017   Today is Saturday. Friday, we had an uneventful day. Nurse Carrie from Kindred Hospice came about 1:30 P.M. She lives in Spanish Trace. She saw Nell's eyes watering and said we ought to treat the watering and the redness as pink eye. She had a prescription called in and I began giving her drops about 5:00 P.M. and again last night (Fri) about 9:00 P.M. Now, this morning, I gave her eye drops after I showered and dressed her. She ate (or drank) an Ensure, a glass of orange juice with her pills. A spoonful of Miralax was dissolved in the orange juice. I am playing in a golf tournament sponsored by Fairhope Baptist Church, invited by a former church member and paid by him. I will leave about 10:00 and return about 7:00 P.M. Laura, one of our church member friends will be the caregiver for the day.

I was gone for 9 hours. All went well with Laura, a church member, and Nell. I put Nell to bed when I got home.

5/1/2017   May is here and I am still healthy, although I had a little food poisoning that I fought for several days, and then had pain in my stomach due to diverticulitis. I took Miralax and amoxicillin after several meals and the pain has subsided.

Today is Monday. We had a terrible thunderstorm last night and the electricity went off, and my breathing machine went off also. I did not sleep well. Nell would roll over toward me, and grab my arm to pull it over to her. I hold her and she seems to respond, by trying to cuddle closer. That is the only affection that is evident in her life now. Although when I came home from golfing Saturday and came in the house, I believe I detected a slight emotional response that she was glad I was home with her. It was just momentary, and then she directed her attention back to the television. But at night there is a desire on her part to hug and be close. I assume that it is her desire to hug me, but it may be anyone. She might need some assurance that someone is taking care of her.

This day has been troublesome. Nell has not looked good. Her eyes were droopy, more than usual. Her ability to walk has been harder. She is very unbalanced and takes very short and slow steps. I felt that she would collapse on the floor at the next step. I have to be so cautious in walking her. She did eat her Ensure very good. She would only eat about three bites of ice cream.

The nurse, Kim, came today and said that all Nell's vitals were very good. Her oxygen level is getting lower, and she made the comment that we might have to put her on oxygen in the near future. Nell went to the toilet after I got her up from her nap. When I changed her Depends, I noticed she was having her feminine issues again. I took her into the shower and cleaned her up. It was a difficult experience.

5/2/2017   Tuesday. I got up to get ready for my Wednesday Senior Choir and nurses aid to come shower Nell. Then it came to my realization that it was Tuesday. I showered Nell and dressed her. She had evidence of feminine issue again, and had an accident I needed to clean. I fed her and all was well. She sat out on the patio while I worked in the yard for about two hours. Then I took her in the house and fed her lunch. When I changed her before her nap she had an accident again and evidence of her feminine issue which needed attention. She napped for two hours and I woke her. I tried to get her to walk to the shower with me to wash her, but her legs just collapsed, and I sat her in the chair in the living room. I waited some time to see if she could walk. I walked her to the bedroom and her legs stiffened to where she could not walk. I picked her up under her arms and sat her in the bedroom chair. We watched the movie Key Largo from about 4:00 to 6:00 P.M. I got her ready for bed. When I took her to the toilet, and removed her Depends she had another accident and cleaned her with evidence of feminine issues again. I got her out of the mess, dressed her for bed, and sat her in the bedroom chair until I cleaned the area.

But with all that, Nell had a good demeanor all day. She had a slight grin all day. Her eyes were so blue. She did not desire to sleep the last few days during the day. She seemed more alert and looked around. One day she looks droopy, awful. The next day she looks alert. In all cases she never says a word. She hasn't spoken in months, not a word to me. Not a word in a long time.

Well, tomorrow is Wednesday, the nurses aid will come and shower and dress Nell. I will take her to E.A. Roberts until after lunch, and then I meet the appointment with the doctor concerning my diverticulitis and Blue Cross annual examination.

5/3/2017   Wednesday started off with a terrible mishap. While making breakfast and feeding Nell at the same time, when I was in the kitchen, she fell off her chair at the breakfast table. Her seat was still on the chair, legs under the table, and head touching the floor. Her face was red and a terrified look on her face. She must have been there, at least, for 30 seconds before I noticed.

I took Nell to E.A. Roberts today, while I rehearsed with the senior choir. Laura Herrington, the Administrator at E. A. Roberts called me and told me that they could not take care of Nell any longer. She was past the stage of Alzheimer's that they care for. She said they could not communicate with her, and she was getting so weak in her legs it was difficult for several of them to get her out of a wheel chair on the potty. Today, her Depends were dry, but when she stood up to sit on the potty, she had feminine issues again. I was not going to argue with them about the need for care at this stage also, but they have been so nice to Nell and I, that I didn't want to leave their acquaintance, with any negative feelings. I brought her home and walked very carefully taking her into the bedroom chair. No more help from E. A. Roberts. Now, any time I can get away, I will have to pay for a caregiver to come in.

5/4/2017   Thursday. Today Melissa comes to shower Nell. Kindred Hospice sent a shower chair for Nell to sit in while she showers and dresses. I will observe how she does this, because I will have to shower Nell on Friday, Saturday and Sunday.

I was going to take Nell to get her hair trimmed and pick up a prescription at Walgreens, but Nell could not walk. We started and her legs stiffened, and could not walk. I was able to get her to a chair, and she stiffened as I sat her in the chair. That was about 4:00 P.M. I waited until daughter, Carrie came about 5:15 with my prescription and she helped me get Nannie ready for bed. I put her on the chair in the bedroom and put a movie on television for her to watch. She did manage to give Carrie a small brief smile.

I cannot plan to go anywhere because Nell may not be able to stand and walk to get into the car. Today, she looked very listless and unattentive to the TV when she was watching it. She just looked away, and layed her head on her shoulder and stared at the door or floor, or whatever.

5/5/2017 Today, I am planning on playing golf with some men from Dauphin Way Baptist. A woman from Knight's Daycare is coming to stay with Nell, in that I cannot take her to E.A. Roberts anymore. It will cost me more to pay for the caregiver than the cost of golf, and lunch. However, this takes my mind off of my daily emotional relationship with Nell in her Alzheimer's disease.

We played golf at Whispering Pines today. I scored an 86. I shot my age in a very windy day. Angela was supposed to be here at 0800. She called about 7:45 A.M., and said she overslept, and said she could be here about 0900. My son-in-law, Calvin was off from work, so he came and sat with her till Angela came. When I got home, she was very apologetic and swore not to let that happen again. Rhee, the housekeeper was supposed to come and clean today, and had a sick child and could not make it today. She has not called as yet, at 6:30 P.M. to reschedule.

Angela seemed to do a good job in caregiving. Nell was at ease watching TV, with Angela sitting beside her touching her when I came in the house. I put her to bed about 6:30 P.M. She was able to stay on her feet. When I changed her Depends there was a little evidence of her feminine issue when I put on the Depends.

5/7/2017 When I was praying this morning (in the closet), The Spirit prompted me to pray in a thankful manner for health to continue to care for Nell. He prompted me to pray for Nell's well-being today, so I could give her good caregiving. She has been weak in the legs off-and-on the last week. Today she walked from the bedroom, with help, to the living room fairly strong, but slow. She is very sleepy. I fed her chocolate Ensure and gave to her the morning pills she is to take. Caregiver Andrea is coming to be with Nell, while I go to worship.

5/8/2017   Monday, Nell did very good. She was strong enough for me to take her to get her hair trimmed. Carrie came to put her to bed while I went to represent Nell at her Murphy class of 53 alumni dinner. She slept well last night.

5/9/2017   Tuesday, I put Nell out front while I mowed the lawn. She seemed strong enough to walk small distances in the house and to the porch. I am disappointed in the family help and concern for Nell and my well-being as caregiver. I do feel quite neglected and alone in the daily care. I need to talk to family and tell them what is going on with Nell, and it seems like I have to initiate a phone call to feel connected. I know family feels all is well when I don't call for help. But I do feel connected with God, and I do pray that God would increase my faith, at times it is weak.

5/10/2017   Wednesday; today, I am going to join up with the senior choir to sing at Palm Garden Nursing home. Knight's Sitting Service, Adrian will be here at 10:00 A.M. to sit with Nell. Nell got up very sleepy and weak in the legs this morning. I fed her Ensure and orange juice with her pills. Melissa is giving her a shower and dressing her now. I am grateful for Kindred Care Hospice who provides the aid to come each day and shower her.

Adrian took good care of Nell. She changed her Depends and later, Nell went to the toilet, and Adrian put on new Depends. When I got home about 2:00 P.M., Nell was laying down for a nap. I got her up about 3:15 P.M. and we sat out on the front porch for about an hour. I gave her some ice cream. She ate a couple of small scoops. I got her ready for bed about 6:00 P.M. and sat her on her bedroom chair. I will get her up from her chair and put her in bed about 7:00 P.M. She was walking a lot better today, and appeared more alert today.

5/11/2017   Thursday. Nell was quite alert when I got her up today. Melissa didn't come to shower Nell today. When I got her up, I showered and dressed her and fed her Ensure. She sat outside while I did some work on the front lawn while it was fairly cool. We went inside when Kim, the nurse, came. Kim informed me that Nell was doing so good this week, that she would only come one day a week, until things changed. It disturbed me to say that she was doing so good, when on the other hand E.A. Roberts said she was doing so bad, she could not come back to E. A. Roberts again.

I talked to Area Agency on Aging who was giving $200.00 a month for Nell's care at E. A. Roberts and said they would continue giving that amount for daycare at home. I believe the amount is $600.00 a quarter.

5/12/2017   Friday. It is about 11:30 A.M. and since Nell got up this morning, she drooped her head over and slept. I took her out front, and she slept. After about an hour I took her in the house, and she slept. I have tried to wake her and get her alert, but to no avail. Nell slept most of the morning. I fed her lunch and layed her down for a nap, which lasted for about 1 ½ hours. I got her up after Mitchell (Grandson) and Emily(-girl friend) got here so they could talk to Nannie. Nannie kind of lit up for a moment, then settled into her regular look. She just looked at the TV. She showed no more emotion of seeing Mitchel. We went for a ride in the car to the drugstore and Nell seemed to perk up and stayed awake and watched several movies before I put her to bed. Later in the afternoon, Nell was alert. But the morning hours she mostly slept.

5/16/2017   Tuesday. Last night when I got into bed, I laid close to Nell and put my arm around her, and said, "I love you." Nell has not said but one word the last six months. She responded in a guttural, kind of mumbled word to say, "I love you." I was astounded. That is why I think a spouse should sleep with their wife or husband who has Alzheimer's. I think at night sleeping beside your spouse, you communicate more by touching, hugging and holding one another more than all the activities of the day.

5/18/2017   This is Thursday. I went to play in a golf tournament today. Caregiver came at 7:00 A.M. Kindred Hospice came at 8:00 and housekeeper came at 9:00. The aid called about a possible UTI. I will follow up on that tonight. I have been in contact with the nurse from Kindred Hospice and their doctor. No medicine prescribed. She seems alright at 5:00 P.M. Seemingly, no discomfort and she can't speak to tell me if there is a problem.

5/19/2017   Friday. The nurse Kim came today to check on Nell's possible Urinary Track Infection and said, she didn't think she was infected. Nell sat out front for awhile and we went down to Rotolos, an Italian restaurant and we sat outside and I ordered some food to go. While we waited I fed her the Ensure I brought for her lunch. I ate a part of my Calzone, and we left. Nell was tired. When we got home she took a nap for about two hours. I took her to the bathroom to change her Depends, and she had an accident. I had to put her in the shower and clean her and put new Depends on her. I then brought her into the living room and she sat in her chair and watched a movie. She slept off and on during the movie. She seems very listless today.

5/21/2017   Today is Sunday. Yesterday, Nell got up and she could not awake. She walked asleep. I could not get her eyes open. Her head was bowed down. She could hardly walk. This morning was different. She got up and her eyes were wide open and alert. She started walking as good as she has walked in a long time. She held her head up. She drank her Ensure good. After she ate I sat her down in her chair, and soon she bowed her head and went to sleep. The caregiver came and took care of her while I went to worship. She did good, and when I got home Nell was taking a nap. After worship, I go to lunch somewhere, in order to have a peaceful meal, not interrupted to feed Nell a sip at a time of her Ensure. That is not a big trouble, but it is good to enjoy a meal.

It is now 7:00 P.M. I just put Nell to bed. She sat in her chair most of the afternoon and watched the golf match with me, where Billy Hoeschel won in a play-off. She did very good except, at various times, she would lean forward as if she was having a pain in her stomach, or in her back. I rubbed her back and rubbed her stomach. She seemed to get some relief from that. But she went to bed and seemed comfortable.

5/22/2017   Monday morning, Melissa showed up at 0800 to shower and dress Nell. I leave the front door open knowing she will be here at that hour. She opens the door and the security door alarm rings and she comes in and says, "How yall."

Last night we went to bed about 7:00 P.M. and the movie *Love is a Many Splendored Thing* came on. Nell seemed to be watching it with some interest. It ended about 8:30 P.M. I turned the TV off and Nell turned over toward me and threw her arm and leg over on me. It was an affectionate manner, that I believe she was trying to express her love to me even though she could not talk. She expresses her love in the only manner she could. I was thinking that we have been through 62 years of many experiences, in the military, in business in California after the military service, then in college and seminary. We ministered together at Cypress Shores Baptist Church and at Dauphin Way Baptist Church. So many experiences together, faded in our memories of long ago. I started talking about various events in our lives to remind her of them. I said, "I know you cannot talk, but I know you can hear. Rather or not you can understand, I don't know, but you can hear." Then I reminded her of many things that took place in our lives. She seemed to acknowledge what I was saying, by moving her arm over me and holding me, as if to say, "I remember those things." I said to her, "True love is a many splendored thing, between you and me for 62 years." She moved her arm over me in a manner, I think, that said to me, "yes."

This morning when I woke her to get her up she looked at me, like, "Who are you?" with a searching, strange look, and kind of fearful.

5/23/2017   Tuesday, raining outside. Last night as I was getting Nell ready for bed, I stood her by the wash basin and she fell away from me and I caught her before she hit the floor hard. I broke her fall, and she landed gently on the floor. This morning I got her up about an hour later than usual. I put her on the potty, and when I went in a few minutes later she had fallen sideways and was leaning against the wall. Melissa came about that time and helped her stand to take a shower. She finally put her on the chair in the shower. Nell's eyes were matting again. I will put some eye drops in her eyes after she showers.

5/24/2017   Wednesday, and Nell had a hard time waking this morning. I guess I should have let her sleep past 7:00 A.M., her regular time. She did not wake up until I walked her to the potty. Melissa came a little late and I put her in her chair and fed her, and Melissa came about 8:20 A.M. and showered her. She dressed her and brought her to the living room to her chair and she went to sleep, and I woke her up about 10:00 A.M. I took some Banana/Strawberry muffins to Carrie and Laurel at State Farm and took a little drive and returned about 12:00 P.M. I fed her and laid her down for a nap. I got her up about 2:00 P.M. She sat in her chair and went to sleep again. I put a movie on the TV, and she watched it for a moment and went back to sleep. Her eyes are very droopy.

5/25/2017   All went well on this Thursday. Melissa came and showered Nell, and Andrea came to be with her while I went to the Veteran's Home in Bay Minette with the Dauphin Way Baptist Church senior choir, The Silvertones, to sing. I also gave a Memorial Day devotion. I went to eat with the Silvertones at Streeter's Restaurant in Bay Minette and then visited Nephew Glen, and family at Stockton. Had a good visit with them. When I left the Restaurant, I had a numbing pain up my left arm. I know that this is sometimes a sign, along with other signs for a heart problem. I have had a numbing feeling in my fingers for some time, and went to the doctor to have him look at it for the possibility of Carpel Tunnel. He gave me a cortisone shot. I don't think it helped much, but I am watching the numbness in my left arm and if there are other signs, I will go to the emergency room.

5/29/2017 Memorial Day. We left Mobile on Saturday morning and had an uneventful trip to Kim's Lakehouse, near Huntsville. We have had several good days on the lake watching grandson-in-law, Randy and the great grandkids fishing (Kids, being Bryce, Brodie, Brooklyn along with grand daughter Britanie and daughter Kim also. They caught two little fish about 6" long. Nell has been no trouble. We are going to eat lunch shortly and I will put her on the bed for a nap.

We went home from the Lakehouse to Mobile on 6/3/2017 Saturday/

6/4/2017 Today, is Sunday, almost a week since I have posted. Nell has had a good week. She has walked fairly well this week. Although, she had a tendency to sleep when she sat down. Last night, she had a deep sleep and at times she stopped breathing, then would pick up the breathing with deep breaths. I got her up and fed her this morning, but did not shower and dress her. I am going to let Andrea earn her caregiving salary and do that when she comes at 0930.

I was laying beside Nell last night and tried to think of the many good times in our 62 years together, but the problems of the moment were too much. All I could remember were the problems of the moment, of the day, of the last several years of Alzheimer's disease.

6/5/2017   Monday and all is well after Nell has been fed, showered, dressed, and is taking a nap about 10:00 A.M. Although I got her up at about 6:15 A.M. this morning because she was wide awake. She seemed quite alert, and walked to the bathroom with help. But Melissa said she was too wobbly and unsteady to have her stand during her shower, so she sat Nell on her chair.

6/6/2017   Tuesday, D-Day. The invasion of Europe to free France from the Nazi's during WWII.

Nell began her day as usual. After she was all showered and fed, she took a nap.

6/10/2017   Nell slept so much on Friday. I tried to get her to sit out front, and she would sleep. When I sat her in her chair to watch television she would sleep. I took her to the back patio to feed her Ensure for her evening meal. It was Butter Pecan flavor. I asked Nell if she liked Butter Pecan. Nell has not said a word in six months, and she just blurted out with good diction, "I like Butter Pecan." I was astonished. That is all she would say. No more words.

6/11/2017   I worked out in the yard this morning. I sat Nell on the front porch so I could keep my eye on her. We visited with Laurel on her first day back from her trip to Alaska. Nell and I went to Café Del Rio, a Mexican restaurant on the Causeway. Nell did well. I pushed her in her wheelchair, into the restaurant and up the elevator. We sat in the water side to view the water and the swamp. She enjoyed looking at the scenery and the people. She likes to look at people. We spent the afternoon at home watching the College Baseball Super regional ball games. Nothing else on after the St Jude Golf Tournament in Memphis.

6/18/2017   Nell would not open her eyes to go to the bathroom this morning. I put her housecoat on after she went to the toilet. I left for church and Andrea was getting her ready for a shower and to dress her. All was well during the morning. When I got back after church, her eyes were droopy and tired to the point it worried me. This was different than at any other time. I got worried that she could be gone at any moment. There was just no response of life in her eyes, like a film was over them. I am concerned, and fearful that her days, her hours are near.

6/21/2017 There has been a confusion as to who was to be here this morning to shower Nell. Melissa has an issue in her neck which causes pain. Shantel, the hospice caregiver, finally came about 9:00 A.M. She is scheduled to be here Thursday through Monday, Not the weekend however.

Today, Nell has been sleepy more than at any time in the past. It is 5:30 P.M. I will probably put her to bed earlier than her usual time of 7:00 P.M.

6/22/2017 Shantel, the Hospice aid, came about 8:15 A.M. this morning and showered Nell. Nell seemed to be a little more alert, but after her Ensure and shower, she was brought into the living room and sat in her chair and went to sleep. The shower tires her out. It is raining outside today, so we will probably not drive anywhere today. Besides, it is very difficult to get her in and out of the car.

I am feeling good, especially, when someone comes and showers Nell and dresses her. That is a problem for me, even though it is not a difficult chore. For some reason I find it a burden to shower and dress her and afterwards, I will admit it was not a burdensome chore, but the next time I prepare to do it, it is a psychological difficult thing to think about doing. Not difficult to do. But it is the same with most of the other housekeeping chores. I dislike doing the washing and folding clothes. I find that mopping the ceramic floor is a psychological difficult thing for me to think about doing. After I do them, I realize that the washing, folding, and mopping was not that hard, and I am ashamed to let some mind roadblock keep me from doing them with ease of mind. It is just hard to do anything except ministering to Nell. That is not easy but does not cause me any problems, except I wish I could do more and keep her more alert mentally and physically. I don't like to see her just sleep. It is not so much a burden to care for Nell as it is all the other chores, even cooking my meals.

6/23/2017   Thursday night I got Nell into bed; tucked her in; put the board barrier up so she would not fall out of bed. Then later, I came to bed and leaned over to her and gave her a hug and said, "I love you." I do this every night. She lays there with her eyes open looking at TV. I don't know what she understands. Sometimes in an emotional scene, I will detect a tear running down her cheek, so I assume there is some comprehension. So, I turn on Turner Classical Movies during the day and evening for her to watch. Nell has not spoken but one small phrase for at least six months. But when I said, "I love you," she responded with difficulty and a kind of "mush mouth," attempt to speak, saying: "I love you." It startled me and pleased me immensely. We went to sleep about 8:30 P.M. I woke up about 2:15 A.M. and could not go back to sleep. So I got up and read. It was on my mind that when I got Nell ready for bed, that her nose was running, and a small brown matter was in the runny nose. When I leaned over and kissed her and told her "I love you," there was an unusual odor that came from her head area. Her eyes were watery when I put her to bed, so I put some eye drops in her eyes. I think that this was a concern and kept me from going back to sleep. So, after reading for several hours I have come to make these comments in the diary. I am going to make some pancake batter and then rest my eyes before I take a walk and come back to do my devotions and prayer before I get Nell up.

6/26/2017   Last night (Sunday), I put Nell to bed, and tucked her in, and told her I loved her. She responded with a very clear, "I love you." During the day we sat on the back patio and listened to Christian music, and I talked to her about our early marriage, and we had a devotion and prayer. Later in the day we were watching a movie and it had a little church with the people singing some old familiar hymns and Nell got emotionally involved. I believe during the day, a lot of events were brought to her mind that recalled her long term memory. I think her brain was awakened a little during the day and it caused a response to say, "I love you." My opinion on why she spoke these words. Now other days we have conversation but she does not awaken mentally like she did when she said last night, "I love you," when I put her to bed.

Tonight when I put her to bed, I sat her on the potty first before I put her night gown and Depends on her. I got to thinking in recent thoughts about my caring for Nell in all kinds of ways, and one of them was cleaning her after going to the toilet. I got to thinking, that I do this so often (almost daily) that it is almost as if I was doing this to myself. It doesn't bother me as it did when I first started cleaning her.

6/29/2017   Thursday. Nell is about the same today. She was alert when I got her up this morning and helped her to the potty. I fed her before the aid came and now she is dressed and sitting in the living room watching TV. I took her outside to the front porch for about an hour. Yesterday, two ladies from the church came and sat with Nell while I went to the doctor to take the stiches out of my Carpal Tunnel surgery. I am meeting A friend for lunch today, and Andrea is coming to sit with Nell from 11:00 to 3:00 P.M. Della Sanchez is coming to our house for a visit from the Area Agency on Aging at 10:00 A.M.

Nell had a bruise with a cut on the top of her hand on the right wrist. I surmise it happened on the plyboard barrier, that is set in the side of her bed so she won't fall out. I think she swung her hand over the barrier and it cut her. I began putting a blanket over the barrier to avoid any hurt.

6/30/2017   Friday. Played golf today and Lynn and Linda were Nell's caregivers. When I returned Linda told me that

Nell had her feminine issues again. I called the Hospice Nurse. She came and looked at Nell and determined it was like the issue she had several months ago. She consulted with the hospice doctor and determined that we continue to give her the medicine that was a hormonal medicine which should help. The nurse, Jan, cleaned her and put on fresh Depends.

7/1/2017   Saturday morning Nell got up and had no physical problems. I showered, and dressed her. Nell seemed to be ok when I awakened her. She did not have any feminine issues overnight and I showered her and dressed her. Then I took her to the breakfast table and fed her. I put her in her chair and she took a nap. She is always ready to take a nap after she does all those little chores in getting up in the morning. After she napped for awhile, I got her ready and we took a drive over to the Malbis shopping area. The traffic was terrible going east and west on I-10. Finally, when I got over there, I found out that I left my wallet at home. But I do put several credit cards in a big business wallet in the car, in case of emergencies, and also to lighten my own carrying wallet. So I pushed Nell around and finally ate at California Dreaming. We came back about 3:00 P.M., and I laid Nell down for a nap. I write these little notes of our day, because I don't know if this will be our last Saturday trip to a shopping mall or not. It is good to know the Journey of Nell's timeline of her lack of ability to do things. I remember when we would go and walk hand in hand and she would also eat. Now she can't chew food at all and walks very short distances. I bring her Ensure, and wheel her in a wheel chair. I fed her Ensure before we went into California Dreaming and when I ate, I fed her a small chocolate milkshake. We had a good time. She seemed to enjoy it. She likes to look around at all the people, so I get a table by the entrance, so she can see people as they come and go

7/4/2017   Today is the fourth of July, Independence Day. All last night into the waking hours of this day, I have felt depressed in my stomach and mind. It's as if God has abandoned me to my situation. I feel bad, that in Nell's Alzheimer's I feel God has abandoned her and is leaving her here on earth to suffer such indignities. She doesn't deserve this. She has always been dedicated to God, and lived a kind, loving manner and was a great helpmeet to me as a pastor in a Baptist Church, and toward the end of our ministry, just when we could enjoy our lives together with not any regular responsibilities, she got this disease. At times I almost lose my faith. I know the devil is putting me through temptations to turn my back on Him. Nell, doesn't know what is going on. I can question God on her behalf, and it puzzles me, and hurts my heart for her.

7/5/2017   It is already the fifth of July, Wednesday. Last night as I was preparing Nell for bed I put her on the toilet and she had an accident, so I put her in the shower and washed her off. She could hardly get out of the shower, she was so weak in her legs. I sat her in the bathroom chair and dried her and dressed her for bed. She scooted down in the chair to where her seat was off the edge. I tried to get her stand up, or if she fell on the floor I would not be able to get her up from the floor by myself. Even getting her up from the chair in that position was hard to do. If she didn't help with her legs, weak as they were, I couldn't have done it. If that experience repeats itself, in a regular way, I will not be able to take care of Nell. If she falls and hurts herself, I will be upset. If she breaks a bone, it would be awful. I might have to consider putting her in a nursing facility, for her good and mine. I have tried to stay away from that. It is getting harder to keep her safe.

Today, things have been a lot better. I took Nell to Super Cuts this morning and had her hair washed and cut. She did very well. I walked her in to the chair where they washed her hair and dried it. They cut it and shaped it. She walked to the car and we returned home. She did very well. Her legs were not weak like they were last night.

7/6/2017   Today (Thursday), Nell got up and was somewhat wobbly in her walking. Last night we went to dinner with family at a seafood restaurant on the Causeway. She did good. I fed her before I left, with Ensure. She also had a milkshake at the restaurant. We got home and I got her in bed about 9:30 PM. This morning the aid showered her and told me that she was very wobbly and she sat her on her chair to dress her. This morning, Della Sanchez, from Area Agency on Aging is coming to visit us. A golfing friend is bringing lunch and visiting with Nell and me.

7/8/2017   This has been a difficult Saturday morning. Nell could not hardly stand when I got her up this morning. It was difficult to walk her into the toilet area. I had to put her into the shower chair to give her a shower, because she was so weak on her feet. I got her out and sat her in her chair outside of the shower, and dressed her while she sat in the chair. Everything was so difficult because Nell was so weak. I put her in the wheel chair and pushed her to the toilet. I took her to the back patio and fed her. All she wanted to do was sleep. I had a hard time feeding her with her head on her chest. But I was able to feed her all of her Ensure. I can wake her and hold her head up. But this is just for a few seconds. She drops her head again in a few moments. It is frightening for me. I think her heart will just stop in a few moments. Or she will go into a state of unconsciousness and just stay in a sleeping condition.

On 7/8/2017 when I told Nell I loved her as we prepared to sleep and the lights were turned off, she replied with just a slight noise from her throat, and not from her lips. I do not believe she can use her vocal chords. Last night as I was talking to Carrie on the phone, I wanted her to get her children to come to Homecoming at Cypress Shores Baptist. I told her I was trying to get in touch with Billy and Anita to also attend. After our conversation I went to take care of Nell and she had tears in her eyes. I think she could understand what was going on. Or maybe the name Cypress Shores triggered some feelings that brought forth tears. She always thought we should have stayed at Cypress Shores when I retired from the pastorate there. After some time at Dauphin Way, she was glad we became members there.

7/11/29017   Tuesday. I am playing golf with some men from the church at Whispering Pines Golf Course in Mississippi today. I will leave the house at 0800. Andrea will stay with Nell. Shantel will come and shower and dress Nell. I try to take care of myself as Nell's caregiver. Hopefully, in the long run, I will be healthy enough to take care of her and not have to put her in a nursing home. Since Saturday, she has been sleeping a lot and her legs have become weaker. I have pushed her in the wheel chair around the house more the last few days, than I have in the past. There has been a slight lack of ability to swallow. Yesterday, I had a French Fry, and I gave her a bite. She kept that fry in her mouth for at least five minutes, and did not hardly chew it, as if she liked the fry but forgot how to chew it.

7/12/2017   Wednesday, I got Nell up and she was walking with a little more stability this morning. The aid, Shantel showered her and dressed her. I put Nell in her chair and she is watching Television.

7/13/2017   Thursday went alright, except the aid did not call until 1:45 P.M. to tell us she was on her way to Shower Nell. I told the aid that I had showered her about 9:00, and told her if she couldn't get here at our house to shower Nell by 9:00, not to come that day. A golfing friend came about 10:30 A.M., and brought lunch from where he lives in Pensacola and left about 1:30 P.M. We had a good lunch and visit. When I got Nell ready for bed, I kept wiping her runny nose, and when I began to brush her teeth, she threw up about a half cup of mucous with some curdled milk, looking stuff. It could have been the vanilla ice cream I gave her about 3:00 P.M. and it came up at about 7:30 P.M. I gave her chocolate Ensure for supper, but I didn't see any of that come up. I put her to bed and gave her a pill to help stop her feminine issue. She went to bed and went right to sleep even though she had slept a good portion of the day.

7/14/2017   I tried to wake her up on Friday morning about 7:00 A.M., so I could feed her early. I tried to wake Nell up to have her breakfast, before the aid arrived to shower her. But I was unable to wake her, and I called Carrie and Bill. I called the nurse to come and check her out. Before the nurse came Laurel came by and she finally gently waked her. When the nurse got here at the house, she checked her out and said her vitals were all good. The caregiver Shantel arrived and took Nell to the toilet and showered and dressed her, and fed her, because I did not want to feed her until the nurse told me it was alright and she would not aspirate and get into trouble. Shantel left about 2:00 P.M. It is now 3:00 P.M. and Nell is resting in her chair watching television and drinking ice tea when I give it to her.

7/15/2017   Yesterday was an emotional day. I had trouble with Nell's physical condition; trouble in my response to several relationships with medical advice regarding Nell's condition and communication involving it. When I got up this morning I was feeling alone, abused and disrespected. I woke about 2:15 A.M. and remembered that I turned the sprinkler on the previous night at about 7:00 P.M. and at 2:00 A.M. the next morning it was still sprinkling. So when I got up and took care of the sprinkling, I just stayed up. I read my devotions and had prayer. God spoke to me from various devotions and prayer. When I read the devotion for the day out of "124 Prayers for Caregivers," my outlook was changed; my attitude was changed. A phrase from Virginia Satir, "Life is not the way it is supposed to be. It's the way it is. The way you cope with it makes the difference." I didn't cope with it very well yesterday, but today I will change the way I coped yesterday, in the power of the Cross of Jesus Christ. John Baille prayed: "Oh thou whose love to man was proven in the passion and death of Jesus Christ, our Lord, let the power of his cross be with me today. Let me love as He loved. Let my obedience be unto death. In leaning upon His cross, let me not refuse my own; yet in bearing mine, let me bear it in the strength of His."

7/18/2017   Yesterday Nell was hard to awaken, like last Friday, but I was not as shocked, and I took my time and touched and gently shook her. Finally she opened her eyes, but was very weak to walk. Through the day she was alright, but slept most of the day. She did alright as I put her in the car and drove around doing several errands. Now this morning, Tuesday, she was awake at 6:00 A.M., when I went into the bedroom to see if she was alright before I went on my walk. I came back from my walk and she was sound asleep. I had the TV on to the morning, local news. Later, I got her up and took her to the potty, and sat her in her bedroom chair and fed her. Shantel came and showered her about 9:00 A.M. and dressed her. She sat her on the shower chair to give her a shower.

7/19/2017   Wednesday, Nell got up fairly easy this morning, I fed her breakfast (Ensure and orange juice) on the back patio, but after her shower, which followed, all she would do was sleep most of the day, even though she went to the toilet several times. Nell has been sleeping most of the day in a deep sleep where she would hardly open her eyes to sip her Ensure.

7/20/2017   I played in a minister's golf tournament at Rock Creek Golf Course in Fairhope today. I had to leave the house at 7:30 A.M. and got back home at 2:30 P.M. Andrea came at 7:30 to care for Nell. The Nurse and Social Worker came about 1:00 P.M. and told Andrea, the caregiver that her vital signs were good. Tonight when I put her to bed, about 6:30 P.M., she had watery eyes, and I put some drops in them. She did not look good tonight. Her legs were weak and I pushed her in her wheel chair to the bathroom and to the bed.

7/24/2017   It has been several days since I have entered anything in my journal. Since I had Carpel Tunnel surgery on my left hand, it has been difficult to type. So, unless there was an unusual event in our lives I have not felt prompted to make an entry or comment. The only thing, is, that the last several weeks, and more in the last several days, Nell just wanted to sleep. I would try to do things, take her for a walk around the kitchen, or wheel her in the wheel chair to the front or back patio. But when I would stop the chair, she would be right to sleep.

One day, I had to go to Lowes to get some PVC materials to fix the sprinkler system. I would load Nell into the car, which is very difficult. When I got to Lowes, I would leave the engine running to keep it cool in the month of July, and try to quickly go in and get what I needed and return. It was not a good thing to do, because someone could jump in the car and drive off. You can't lock the car with the key in the ignition, but all worked out well.

A couple of nights ago, I woke up about 2:00 A.M. and checked Nell to see if she was covered. She felt cold all over. She was laying on her back, with her mouth open, and she didn't seem to be breathing. I thought to myself, that she has gone to be with the Lord. I thought, "What do I do now?" I could not determine if she had a pulse. I could not feel her heart beat, then she moved her leg, and I was relieved. Yet, in a sense (I feel awful to say it), I had a feeling that I hoped she had gone to be with Jesus. I laid back down beside her and held her close, to warm her and I felt a love for her and regretted my thoughts. Yet I have those thoughts from time to time.

Last night Jonathan, my grandson, came by about 6:00 P.M. with great grandchildren, Ryleigh and Whit to visit us. Nannie was in her chair and they came to greet her. She just looked at them with a kind of screwed up expression. I think she had some thought about the children, and all she could do was to express it in a grimace, or whatever. Nell has not said over two short phrases in six months or more. Before that, the previous six months she was just parroting words someone else said. She immediately turned her attention back to the TV program she was watching. The great grandchildren, so young, Whit in the second grade, and Ryleigh, a four year old, looked at Nannie with such sympathy and sorrow on their faces. Nannie would have loved to hug them and kiss them but had no ability to do that in her Alzheimer's condition. She just loved her children, grands and great grandchildren, and now to see her helplessness in expressing that love is very hurting. The children don't know how to express their affection to their grandmother and great grandmother. They are very standoffish, and unsure how to relate. But I notice that is the way for all her friends who come to visit or acquaintances she sees out in a public place. I think our children, and grandchildren, would rather not see her in this condition, but to remember her as she was, when healthy.

On 7/25/2017 I told Nell, "I love you", as I do each night when I get in bed. She tried to respond and all that came through her lips was a feeble attempt to say, "I love you", with a grunting noise of "harumph rumps." It was beautiful and heartwarming. Last night, watching a movie where the end showed a military man & sweetheart finally come together in a promise to marry and the movie ended with their kissing. Nell showed some emotion with a slight grin. I said to Nell, " That is like you and I when you pinned my wings on me and then you married me in a military uniform." Nell just stared at me. I believe behind those eyes, she remembered, but I did not see any acknowledgement. It was like "I wish I could remember that, or I remember, but was that you?" Or maybe she was not able to move from the movie situation to her own experience at all. She did enjoy the ending of the movie; I could tell that.

7/26/2017 This is Wednesday. After Nell was showered and fed, and the aid put her in her chair, I went out and mowed the lawn. It was fairly cool, with broken clouds that shielded the sun, mostly. She slept through it all. Last night, Nell and I watched a movie before she went to sleep. It had a good love story as the subject. At the end of the long movie, Nell was still attentive. I tucked her in and as I usually do, I told her, "I love you." She mumbled back to me, "harrumph fphumpf." I know she was trying to respond with, "I love you," but that was the best she could do. It was beautiful and heartwarming. She has been sleeping most of the morning. She was hard to wake up this morning. I had to open her eye lids and soon she kept her eyes open by herself.

7/30/2017   Sunday morning as I reflect back on yesterday, Nell was looking alert, and rested after her afternoon nap. I decided to take her for a ride and we went to downtown Mobile to look at her early youth environment. I drove around and showed her a lot of the places she was familiar with as a young person before we were married. I showed her where we met on the town square. I showed her the old building she was familiar with as the 5, 10 cent store, and also where Gayfers and Morrison cafeteria was located. I showed her where the old Cawthorn Hotel was located, and where the Peanut store and old theater is located on Dauphin St. I did not notice any expression or emotion of recognition of anything. She sat in the car, put her foot on the dashboard, and just stared straight ahead, not looking when I pointed things out. When we got home, I fed her and got her into bed. I put a Netflix movie on our TV, and she attentively watched it. I turned the lights out after the TV movie was over and held her close and told her I loved her, but with no response

It is 7:00 A.M. Sunday, and I will get Nell up and feed her before the caregiver Andrea arrives to be with her while I attend worship services and have dinner.

7/31/2017   Monday. I reflect back on yesterday. When I got home from church, Nell was on the couch where the caregiver laid her for a nap. She was awake and her head was turned toward me, as she heard my voice when I entered the room. I went to speak to her and her eyes were dark and staring. She continued looking toward me to her left as she was laying on her back. Staring to her left. Not seeming to look at anything, with no movement of her eyes, just staring. After a hour, she turned her head and slept for about a half hour. Then she turned her head in my direction where I was seated, not looking at me, but in my direction. She again stared without any movement of her eyes. I got her up from the couch, and put her in her chair, so she could watch T.V. The new thing this Sunday in her condition was her seeming dark eyes, just staring. Normally, her eyes are flashing blue, but her eyes became a dark look. Even when I put her to bed in the evening, her expression was blank and dark.

8/1/2017   Evening of Tuesday. I put Nell to bed about 7:15 tonight. She seemed to be sleepy. She weighed 116.4 this morning when she took a shower. She has been loosing weight even though I give her an Ensure three times a day, plus several scoops of ice cream in the afternoon. I am going to try to give her something else in the mid morning hours to see if I can get her stabilized. Maybe I will try Activia. I have in the past and she didn't take to it too well. She looks alert in her eyes but just stares. She does not seem to hear noises, or noises don't arouse her attention. I talked to her this morning at breakfast on the back patio. I looked in to her eyes and she stared into mine. I determined to look into her eyes and keep on talking. She looked into my eyes and did not show any emotion or visible understanding of anything I was saying. After some time she finally looked elsewhere. I hate to verbalize the fact that she looked at me and I looked into her eyes and there was no more response than you would get looking into the eyes of an animal. I say that with affection, not meaning any meanness, but a loving relationship with an animal. When I go to bed at night, I don't know if I will awaken to a live wife, or one who has gone on to God's paradise. I think about this and turn over and hug her with my arm around her and express my love to her. There is no response or reaction emotionally of any kind.

8/3/2017   Last night, watching a movie where the end showed a military man & sweetheart finally come together in a promise to marry and the movie ended with their kissing. Nell showed some emotion with a slight grin. I said to Nell, "That is like you and I when you pinned my wings on me and then you married me in a military uniform." Nell just stared at me. I believe behind those eyes, she remembered, but I did not see any acknowledgement. It was like "I wish I could remember that, or I remember, but was that you?" Or maybe she was not able to move from the movie situation to her own experience at all. She did enjoy the ending of the movie; I could tell that.

Today, I took Nell to Orchid Day Spa and she had a manicure and pedicure. It is difficult getting Nell out of the car and back into the car. But it was worth it to have her fingers and toes trimmed and painted. Afterwards, I drove over to North Mobile Rehabilitation to look over the facility where I now plan to take Nell, while I go on a five night respite at the Gulf in Kim and Pat's condo, Beach Walk. I plan on being alone, and just do what I want to do. I will swim in the pool, or a walk on the beach, go to the restaurant of my choice, read, etc. I don't want to be involved with other people and their desires. I will just go alone.

8/4/2017   Today is Friday. Nell got up fairly easy this morning, and I got her on the potty about the time that Andrea arrived at 8:00 A.M. I have been concerned with the loss of weight Nell is experiencing the last several weeks. She weighs 116 this week. Last week it was 118. So I decided to give her food in some way she would eat it. So today she was fed her orange juice and Ensure at breakfast, Ensure at Lunch and supper. Today Andrea fed Nell Non Fat Yogurt about mid-morning and ice cream in the mid afternoon, and this is beside the Ensure at her meal times. When I came home from golfing, I said "hello" to Nell. She was watching TV, and did not change her expression and continued steadfastly looking at TV, with no recognition. Her eyes did not change from her focus as if she was blind and deaf.

8/5/2017   Saturday morning. Last night I had an unusual dream. It was contemporary, yet it went back many years. I was in the house overnight of a lady in our church. I was not particularly attracted to her. Yet there was something sexual in my thoughts. Then, the scene changes to my getting ready to leave in the morning, and Nell was the central figure in the house and this lady in the church was no longer in the scene. Nell's best high school friend showed up with her sisters, and they were wondering what I was doing at Nell's house all night. The scene switched back and forth between Nell and this (not real attractive) lady in our church. There was thoughts from Nell's friends that there was something sexual happened during the stay there that night, and Nell was acting very smug about it. We never was involved sexually before we were married. It evidently was before we got married, yet this lady in the church was involved in some sexual unfulfilled fantasy in my dream, but one who I am not attracted to sexually, but a nice lady. I think the dream came out of a frustrated sexual life, since Nell got Alzheimers. There has been no sexual life, but not that there was no desire on my part, but not to be unfaithful to Nell with any other person. I just mention this, in case, some male person reads this who is taking care of a wife who has Alzheimer's.

I took Nell to the Bel-Air Mall this morning. I pushed her around so she could look at the shops and the people. I ate lunch at the Chinese restaurant and fed Nell her Ensure. She stayed awake in our drive back home and when we got home I laid her down for a nap. She slept about an hour and a half. I was watching the golf game on TV, and when I put her in her chair, she watched it from moment to moment.

8/6/2017   Sunday morning I took Nell out to the back patio to feed her the Ensure and Orange Juice with Muralax. I had Pandora playing Christian music. I went into the kitchen and when I came back to the patio where Nell was sitting in her wheel chair, she had scooted down, almost off the wheel chair. By the time I got her back on the chair safely, I was in a sweat. I almost called Carrie to come help me. It was difficult because of the recent Carpel Tunnel on my left hand. It was painful to get my hand under her shoulder and try to pull her back up on the chair. Finally, I gave one last big pull, pain or not and got her up. Such is another experience in our day, and this is just the beginning of the day.

I came home from church around 4:30 P.M., today, because of a Men's meeting at the church. After the meeting the men, about ten, gathered around me and prayed for Nell and I. The church has been quite concerned in their praying for Nell and I concerning Nell's Alzheimer's disease, and my caregiving.

In the afternoon, Laurel came to our house to bring me a spaghetti dinner. She greeted Nell, and talked to her, and soon Nell began to "screw" up her face, and a slight amount of tears began to appear around her eyes. I thought it was the eye infection for which I have been treating her. But, when I looked more closely, it was tears. This is the first time I have seen her show any sure outward emotion.

8/7/2017   Monday begins a new week. Shantel will be here about 0830 and give Nell a shower and dress her. Nell was so pitiful last night. She just looked tired and when I put eye drops in her eyes, she just held her eyes tightly closed, and it was difficult getting the drops in her eyes. We watched a nice movie and she was attentive. When I turned the lights out, I leaned over and put my arms around her and held her close, and told her I loved her. There was no response from her as is the usual case. Every morning when I come to get her up, she is laying on her back, with her mouth slightly open, and no movement, and it appears as if she is gone from this life. I am torn between two emotions: one, is that I hope she has gone to be with the Lord, and two, that she would wake up and be alert for the day. I feel like a hypocrite. I hold her closely at night, and have an emotion of love in my heart for Nell, and yet, hope she goes to be with the Lord during the night. It is difficult to sort through and explain my feelings. I think, "Is this just being selfish?" Then I try to justify my thoughts that the Lord take her to be with Him, and think, "This is what is best for Nell? There is a lot of guilt in my heart for thinking this. This morning, (7:00 A.M.) she is still in bed, and soon I will get her up, and express my love for her in taking her to the potty, and getting her robe on her, feeding her and taking care of her the best I can. Then Shantel comes and gives her a shower, and dresses her. We begin another day. It is such a relief to have Shantel come to get her ready for the day. I did this for quite a while, and it was always difficult. Now, I just shower and dress her on Saturdays. Andrea, the caregiver who comes on Sundays, gives her a shower and dresses her. Nell is getting weaker and it is difficult for her to stand in the shower. Even sitting in the chair is difficult. you still have to be alert that she doesn't fall off of the chair.

8/8/2017 Last night, Monday, Nell and I watched a movie in bed. It was a good and sentimental movie that Nell watched all the way through. When it was over, I turned out the lights and leaned over to her and held her close for a few minutes to give her some security. I said, "I love you." She replied with a guttural sound from her throat. I don't believe she can use her vocal chords or tongue or lips. So from her throat she attempted to reply with a, "I love you."

Today, two church ladies, Francis and Patty came to sit with Nell for several hours while I went to the dentist. They sat next to Nell and talked to each other. That is a good visit and care.

8/12/2017 I haven't written anything for several days. Nell did not show any difference in her health for several days. Today, Saturday, I took her shopping at the Malbis Shopping Mall in Baldwin County. I pushed her around in the wheel chair and into Kirklands. She always liked to shop in Kirklands in Mobile, so I took her in the store. She showed no interest.

Did not look at anything, At times her head bowed down and I had to pick it up to look. We went to California Dreaming for lunch. I fed her the Ensure I brought for her, and I ate a salad & Chicken sandwich. I brought more than half of it home for supper. I brought her home and took her to the bathroom and she hardly needed to have her Depends changed. I laid her down for a nap, where she slept for several hours.

It will be a test for me to go to the Gulf for a week, while Nell goes to a nursing home. I am somewhat at ease with Andrea going to the center twice a day for several hours checking up on her. I don't feel good about myself as I relate to Nell at times. She shows no response to anything that I do for her, which I do not believe she knows to respond. When another female comes to my home, I almost feel like turning my attention to this women, because Nell does not seem to be alive, or is no company to me by any response anyway. The Lord says, "There is no temptation that comes to us that He will give a way to escape," and in the Lord's prayer we are told that when we pray "Lead us not into temptation, and deliver us from Evil," He does it, as long as we look to the power of the cross to deliver us. We must flee those temptations. But I admit they are there.

8/13/2017   This is Sunday and we are preparing to take Nell to a nursing home for her to stay there for 5 nights which will be through Friday night the 18th. She is all packed. Today, she seems to be alert.

8/14/2017   Monday, I got Nell up, showered and dressed her. I fed her Ensure and Orange Juice with Mira-lax. I took her to the nursing home about 8:45 A.M. They checked us in the room on the dementia ward about 10:00 A.M. The administration did not get the word, when I checked in on Thursday, that I would bring Nell about 9:00 A.M. They were not ready, because they said they were not informed of that time by the person who checked me in Thursday. I was somewhat in a hurry to check her in because I wanted to attend David

Roan's funeral at Radney Funeral Home. After the funeral, I had lunch with several men from the church and then drove to the Gulf and moved in to Kim's condo, the Beach Walk. I arrived about 2:30 P.M.

I felt like a traitor when I took Nell in to the Nursing Home, knowing that Nell had often told me never to put her in a nursing home if she ever got disabled. I felt like I was doing something behind her back, sneaking her in and then my sneaking out, and leaving her there, with no ability to say anything or to disagree with what I was doing. I don't know what is going on behind her eyes. There didn't seem to be any emotion in them, or any kind of reaction emotionally. But who knows what is happening in her mind. I felt awful. I hope I am doing what is best in my caregiving for long term health on my part to care for Nell. I want to do what is best, but I don't know if this is healthy for me. Time will tell.

8/15/2017   Nell's first night at the nursing home. I phoned Andrea last night and she told me they took good care of her and Andrea walked her to the solarium during the day. I did not sleep well last night. When you are used to having your partner to touch during the night, it is comforting.

This is the first whole day that Nell has spent in the nursing home. I played 9 holes of golf before I got rained out. I ate lunch at Ruby Tuesdays on a gift card and came home. I read all afternoon and did some typing on a procedure for having a happy family if the family is in the middle of troubles.

8/16/2017   Had a hard time sleeping at the Gulf Tuesday night. I got a call from Carrie this morning. She reported that Calvin went by to visit Nell yesterday and was disappointed in the surroundings. She said he was disappointed and would have taken her home if he had the authority and ability to care for her. I talked to Andrea about Calvin's misgivings. Andrea said that she thought they were doing a good job and feeding her food that they pureed, and that she was eating it. I think I will still go on my plans to take Nell home on Saturday. Andrea said she thought Nell was aware that she was not at her home, or at least, she was aware she was in unfamiliar surroundings.

8/18/2017   Friday. I am home from the Gulf. In the morning (Saturday) I am scheduled to go to the nursing home and pick up Nell and bring her home. It hasn't been good this week. I have missed Nell's presence even though there is no interaction between us. I am just busy taking care of her, and I do that with loving care. I sense her presence and forget she is not here. When I am mowing the lawn, I have to come in the house to check on her and remember she is not in the house. When I wash the clothes and fold and put them up, I think to myself, "Nell will be proud of me putting the clothes up before I go to bed." I am mixed up mentally. It would be a lot easier for me for Nell to be in a nursing home, but I can't live in our house and not have her live in it with me. She may not even know, but I know how she felt about nursing homes, and I know how she loved her home. I feel sick to my stomach about her being at the nursing home, and I am able to bring her home, but I will not bring her home until in the morning.

8/19/2017   It is 2:00 A.M., Saturday morning, and I am up. I cannot sleep, even though I am physically tired from playing golf on Friday. I joined Carrie and Calvin to eat last night at a Thai restaurant in St. Elmo. I enjoyed the fellowship, and evening meal, but missed having Nell with us even though she would only drink Ensure, but she would be with us. I am looking forward to having Nell back home again, so I can tend to her.

Carrie and I went to pick Nell up at the appointed time of 10:00 A.M., and they had not got her up from bed. We waited about 20 minutes for the aids to dress her and get her ready. The head nurse said that no one had told her that Nell would be going home this morning (Saturday). Nell was pitiful. She was so depressed in appearance. She looked at Carrie and I with stares, looked like trying to figure out who that was looking at her, and pushing her in a wheel chair and putting her in the car. Her head drooped over and she went to sleep as we drove home. All she has been doing since I brought her home is sleeping. I have been sitting near her since she has come home and I fed her, and later gave her a small banana smoothie. She looks at me with eyes and a face that is screwed up. The appearance breaks my heart. I keep telling her that she is home. She will get to sleep in her own bed tonight. I believe tomorrow will be a better day for her after she sleeps in her bed and Andrea gives her a shower and dresses her.

I do not feel good today of our experiences in bringing her home after being separated for these past five nights and five days.

8/20/2017 Sunday. This day has been a worry. I could not wake Nell this morning as I usually do. I finally had to pull her out of bed and stand her on her feet before she opened her eyes. I sat her on the wheel chair and took her to the toilet and sat her on the toilet, then got her up and put her housecoat on her. I fed her in the breakfast area, and then Andrea arrived and she showered her and dressed her. When I returned from worship and lunch, Andrea told me that when she took a nap in the morning hours, it was hard to awaken her from her morning nap. Also, after her shower when Andrea was drying her she had an accident before she got to the toilet. That was the fourth time she went to the toilet since I brought her home from the nursing home. I think they gave her too much Mira-lax for her to go to the toilet that many times in a 24 hour period. Then in the afternoon she took a nap and when I got her up and sat her on her chair, she took another nap. In the mid-afternoon I usually give her several scoops of ice cream, but she would not open her mouth to take a bite. I sat beside her and rubbed her feet while I watched the golf game. She would open her eyes once in a while. I looked at her and asked her if she liked me to rub her feet. She just looked at me with no response. I told her that I loved her and she gave a big awkward smile. I was shocked and pleased at her response. But that was it. There was no other sign of communication or emotion. She is still not back to her condition she was in when I took her to the nursing home. I thought she was in heaven this morning when I tried to wake her. When she was napping, I thought she was in heaven. She is not alert as she was when I took her to the nursing home. I think going to the toilet that many times made her more weak and sleepy than usual.

8/24/2017   Thursday. I haven't made any entries in the diary for several days. It has been much the same every day. Nell sleeps most of the time. This morning she got up fairly easy. After she was dressed, she was placed in her chair and slept most of the morning. I waked her several times and tried to give her a little snack, but she would not open her mouth. She just slept. I gave her Ensure for lunch and then laid her down on the couch for her to take a nap. It is 12:15 P.M., and she will sleep until 2:00 P.M. and I will wake her up, change her and take her for a little walk.

8/26/2017   Saturday. My birthday of 87 years. I got Nell up this morning. She was easy to awaken. But she was so weak to get her on her feet. When I tried to shower her, it was difficult to get her into the shower, because she was so weak. I put her in her wheelchair and dressed her. I took her to the back patio to feed her, and she sat there for an hour and listened to Christian hymns on Pandora. I put her in her chair and she mostly slept through the morning hours.

8/28/2017   Monday. Nell had some feminine problems again yesterday, and this morning. I gave her the prescription before bedtime recommended so to not have the problem, Nell has been more alert these last several days. Yesterday, after church services, I went to eat lunch by myself. I got to thinking that soon that this may be a constant experience. Nell cannot go out to eat with me, but, even though she is not able to do anything, and I have to do all to take care of her, she is still company to me. I talk to her, and take care of her, and sleep with her. Her "presence" is company, even though she has not said a word, in months, or given evidence of any kind of response to anything that I do, she is still "present." I missed her when I put her in a nursing home, while I went to the Gulf for a week of respite care. I would miss her greatly, if she was permanently placed in a nursing home, even though I could visit her daily. I know that if the Lord takes her from me, thinking selfishly, I would miss her greatly, even though her residence would be better with the Lord. Her life is just "here." As far as I can determine, she is not aware of her sur-roundings, or recognizes anyone, even me. My heart goes out to her, and my caregiving is not diminished because of her lack of awareness. I am lonely, even though she is next to me in her chair, she gives no company, except she is "present." Yet, if she wasn't there near in a chair I would be more lonely. Conversa-tion is one thing, and a person's presence is another thing. So, a person's presence does not completely take away lonliness. Conversation must be part of one's relationship to take away the lonliness. When we sleep together and she throws her leg over me and I take her hand, she seems comforted. That could not happen if she was in a nursing home.

8/29/2017   Tuesday, Nell got up quite good this morning. She had a little femine issue again. She ate good and after her shower and was dressed she was seated in her chair by Chantel. She sat there for most of the morning. She ate a little amount of smoothie mid-morning and I sat her on the back patio for about a half hour. After lunch, I took her to the bathroom to change her and she had evidence of her feminine problem. I gave her a pill that was prescribed to stop that problem. By the evening she was nearly healed from her problem. She was very tired when I put her to bed tonight about 6:30 P.M.

9/2/2017   Saturday morning. Andrea, the caregiver took care of Nell while I was played golf on Friday. She said

Nell was having her feminine issue again. I gave her a pill of Magestrol about 3:30 P.M. She was still in her problem when I put her to bed. She slept good all night long. It is now 6:00 A.M. in the morning. I got up about 4:00 A.M. Yesterday, I got up about 2:00 A.M. I could not sleep, so I got up. Wednesday, I went to Senior Choir Rehearsal. When I went into the building, I thought it was cold in the building. After choir began, I got a chill. After a while, I began to shake with chills. I left to go home and get under the covers. I heard of people who had nervous breakdowns and I thought I must be having a nervous breakdown. I have had a nervous stomach while I was sleeping and I would wake up with a nervous stomach. So I thought maybe I was having a nervous breakdown. I had a preacher friend in California who had a nervous breakdown and he just collapsed while standing in the church fellowship hall. He never was normal after that. He couldn't do anything. He was actually never right emotionally after that, so I guess I was worried about a nervous breakdown. On the way home from church from Senior choir, I decided to stop at the urgent care facility in Saraland. The doctor told me after he analyzed a urine sample that I had a prostate infection. I began taking an antibiotic about 5:00 P.M. and another about 9:00 P.M. Then another about 12 midnight. By Thursday morning I was not shaking, but I felt weak. I played golf on Friday and shot an 89, even though I was not in the best of shape, but I had a foursome to fill out so I went and played. Even in my sickness I was able to care for Nell. God gives me the ability, love and physical strength to take care of Nell. Even though at times, I look to God to be gracious and merciful to take Nell out of her physical condition, then I try to be honest and think, that is just my selfish spirit. I think it is my fleshly nature that I want God to take away this constant responsibility. But, if it was reversed, I know that Nell would not be selfish, and would take care of me, without those fleshly thoughts. That is just the way she is, or was, as I think she is really not personally with me, in her Alzheimer's.

I married Nell knowing she was 6 years younger than me, and that women usually live longer than their husbands, she would be taking care of me in my old age. Children don't take care of fathers after their mothers die, like they do their mothers, after the father dies. I thought Nell would be my nurse until God chose to take me to Himself in the Paradise of God, but it has turned the other way, and God has given me the ability to be faithful to my responsibilities.

Saturday, in the afternoon after Nell had a nap, I took her into the toilet area to change her and see if she could go to the potty. She went to the toilet and she still had evidence of her feminine issue. I finally got her clean. She had her feminine issue and was looking down, I believe, embarrassed, as I put her in her wheelchair. I lifted her chin and said to her, "I love You." I don't believe she is aware of her surroundings to any extent. I took her on the back patio. It was hard to take her there, but all she did was drop her head and sleep, so I brought her back in the house because it was too warm outside.

9/3/2017   Sunday. Here it is Labor Day weekend. So Sunday Nell and I are making plans to sit around the house again like every other weekend. Everybody else is having family time, enjoying the weekend together. But when you have a family member who has Alzheimer's, that member does not fit in for family fun. That victim doesn't know what is going on, but just to be carried to a chair and sleep, or stare, or watch TV, with (I don't think) no comprehension. So who wants to take care of that problem on a fun day. The regular caregiver, that's who. The family feels more guilty on these days, like Labor Day, or Thanksgiving or Christmas. Those are the toughest days for family. They have family, and Nell is not aware of the day or even cares as far as I can see if she is not with family or anyone else. "Just feed me and keep me clean," I think she would say, if she had the sense to realize, that is the truth of the matter. She is an Alzheimer's victim, but, of course, she can't help it, so we do all that we need to do to make her comfortable in this life as long as we need to. Our hearts go out to her.

She is in bed now on Sunday night at 7:30 P.M. watching TV. She will become disinterested soon and go to sleep. The feminine issue occurred today according to Andrea who took care of her while I went to worship and dinner. This evening she didn't have any evidence of the issue continuing. I walked her out to the back patio this afternoon about 4:00 P.M. for about a half hour. She sat and squirmed in the chair, and so finally I took her back to her chair in the house and propped up her legs. I fed her about 5:30 P.M. and she drank her Ensure to the last drop.

9/4/2017   Labor Day, Nell and I drove to Daphne, and I put her in the wheel chair and rolled her on the Alligator Alley. We ate lunch at a picnic place in Alligator Alley. She drank her Ensure and I ate some chicken nuggets and fries. There was a man sitting on a picnic table nearby. He looked like a homeless man, so I gave him the balance of my chicken nuggets and French fries. He was reading a New Testament, and gave me a testimony. He would have engaged me for some time, but I had to leave. Nell was getting squirmey in her wheel chair. I did some grocery shopping and we came home arriving about 1:00 P.M. I cleaned her and laid her down for a nap. She had evidence of her issue, and went to the potty. I was going to get her up about 3:30 P.M. from her nap but she was too tired, so I let her sleep some more. Her outing got her too tired, although she stayed awake during our complete trip.

9/6/2017   Wednesday. This is Senior Choir Rehearsal day. Andrea comes to take care of Nell, and she also does the washing, folds and puts away the clothes, makes the bed with clean sheets, and I give her an additional $10.00. Nell is still involved in her feminine issue. Since Friday, her issue has been moderate, heavy and slight, but still persisting, even though I have been giving her the medicine Magestrol. Nell has been sleeping lately with her mouth slightly open and looks like she has died. It scares me when she sleeps. She will sleep all the time if I would let her. Once I get her up and set her watching television, she will watch a little. Then, she will stare at the door or some other object, and not pay any attention to the TV. She just doesn't seem to be involved in any way with things in her environment, at times.

9/7/2017 Thursday. Today has been an uneventful day. Andrea came and sat with Nell today, while I played golf, because tomorrow I will be attending a funeral. Today, while I was playing golf, Andrea called to get permission to let her son come and stay with her at our house. He had a bad headache and Andrea needed to have him with her. Nell seemed to be alert all afternoon, and watched TV. She did not sleep. She was easy to put to bed tonight, and still seemed alert while I got her in bed.

9/9/2017 Saturday. I had a hard time waking Nell up today. She was as limp as a wash rag while I showered her and dressed her. I fed her in her chair in the living room, and afterwards she went back to sleep again, until I fed her Ensure for lunch, then she laid down for an afternoon nap.

9/10/2017 Sunday. As I was getting Nell up from the toilet this morning, she was holding the bar while I was getting the wheel chair to put under her, her right leg gave way and she fell between the wall and toilet. When I got her into wheel chair, there was blood on the floor where she dripped from several arm cuts and a leg gash. I got her into the wheel chair and put bandages on three different wounds. I went to Cypress Shores Baptist Church Homecoming today. I attended a meeting at Dauphin Way Baptist Church and did some grocery shopping and got home about 4:30 P.M. Andrea said all went well. She needed to dress Nell's wounds that occurred during the morning toilet time, after she got up from her nap. I don't know what to do tonight to get her to bed, Andrea said she was still limping on her right foot. She may have had a slight stroke.

9/11/2017 Monday. Calvin came and stayed with Nell while I went to the Dauphin Way Baptist Men's Prayer Breakfast. Shantel came and got her up from bed, showered and dressed Nell. When I got home about 8:30 A.M. I fed her the Ensure and orange juice with Mira Lax in it. She slept most of the morning. I got her up after she napped about two hours after lunch and took her to the potty. I put on new pull up diapers. I took her to the patio and gave her a glass full of vanilla ice cream mixed with Almond Milk, a half of a banana and three ice cubes in the milk shaker. She drank most of it. I put a movie on the TV and sat her down to watch it about 3:15 P.M. I went to Nell's Murphy Class of 53 Reunion at Briquettes Steak Restaurant and returned home about 8:20 P.M. Calvin stayed with Nell while I was gone. When I returned home I put Nell to bed. She seemed calm and I was able to get her into her night clothes and lay her down in bed easily.

9/12/2017 Tuesday. I have had trouble getting Nell up, taking her to the potty, feeding and getting her ready for the Kindred Care Aid to shower and dress. She has fallen in the potty area several times when I had her holding the bar, while I reached around to get the wheel chair to put under her. She would stand while I cleaned her and her legs would get so weak, that by the time I was able to get the wheel chair under her she would be so weak, especially in her right leg. She seemed to walk as if it pained her. So today I am not going to get her up until the aid comes, if she comes before 9:00 A.M. If not, then I will have to do the shower and dress her myself. I never know. Shantel came and put her on the potty, showered her and dressed her. Nell was so weak, especially in her right leg. Shantel told me afterwards that she was going to order me a bedside commode because Nell was getting so weak. That I could spray her with shower wash, and dry her with baby wipes; clean her after she goes to the potty, while she is sitting down.

Nell is in the stage now where she is going to be taken care of mostly without using her legs. Maybe just to get up on the floor and put in a wheel chair, and taken to her chair in the living room. Walking is just about out, at least, in the experience of the last several days. Shantel said that Nell was involved in her feminine issue a little today. We tried to weigh her and the closest we could get in her standing on the scales was 110 lbs. The nurse Jan came today and along with Shantel has given me different instructions to care for Nell now that she is getting weak and favoring her right leg in walking. I will begin her morning by putting her on a bedside potty rather than walking her to the toilet. After she goes to potty, I will clean her and put her in her bedroom chair, feed her, and wait for the Aid to come shower and dress her.

9/13/2017   Wednesday. Yesterday nurse Jan from Kindred Care Hospice, came and looked at Nell's vitals and dressed the several wounds Nell got from falling in the toilet area of the bathroom. I told Jan that sometimes Nell seemed to be pouting. I remember her attitude when she was normal, when she would pout. I could tell. Which was very seldom, but I could tell. I told Jan I thought she was angry at me, and at times she would pout. I think she was pouting over letting her fall in the toilet area. I took my hand off of her for just seconds as I turned to get her wheel chair and she fell. That happened twice last week. Her legs were too weak to hold her up long, and she fell. When I told Jan that Nell was pouting, Jan asked her if that was true. Nell screwed up her face and opened her mouth wide as if to say, "yes that is true, I was angry for him letting me fall." We both read that into her expression. It was amusing to see her response.

Hospice sent a hospital bed to help me get her in and out more easily.

Today, when I got her up from her hospital bed she was far too weak to stand, and Shantel put the wheel chair under her immediately, because she was going to fall. Shantel showered her and dressed her. She told me that on Thursday, she was going to bathe her on the potty chair, because she was too weak to shower. It was hard on her to try to keep Nell on her feet to move her from her shower chair to the potty, to dry and comb her hair. So, tomorrow we will go to another stage in caregiving. We will not shower her anymore. I came home from senior choir and lunch, and Andrea told me that she had a difficult time trying to get Nell to the toilet. She was so weak that she could not walk easily. Kindred Care Hospice had a potty chair delivered, so I will use that to get her to bed tonight. No more toilet, in the bathroom, but now a potty by the bed. She has been taking a nap this afternoon. It is now 2:00 P.M. and I will get her up in about a half hour.

9/14/2017 was the first day Nell was bathed and dressed on her bedside potty. It was also the first day I changed her Depends while she laid on the sofa in the living room. These were not the pull-ups, but wrap arounds.

9/14/2017 Thursday. Last night when I was preparing Nell for bed, I put her on the bedside potty for the first time. It looks like this will be a new level in her caregiving, because she is too weak to stand in the toilet area of the bathroom and get her in the wheel chair after she sits on the toilet. This is where she fell twice in about a week. While she was standing, holding the bar, I would reach to get the wheel chair and she would collapse. So, last night I put her on the potty chair beside the bed, and she sat on the potty. I cleaned her and put her gown on her. Then I put her Depends on her legs, stood her up and pulled them up and put her on the bed and laid her down. I think this is the safe way, and it will be a whole new procedure in putting her to bed at night. I will wait for the Kindred Care Aid to get her up in the morning to put her on the potty chair, and then on to the wheel chair and shower her and dress her. Or, she might bathe her while she is on the potty chair and dress her there. Then put her on the wheel chair and take her to her chair in the living room. Kindred Care said they were going to send an aid on Saturday mornings now to get her up and dress her. (They never did. I did it on Saturday.) Andrea, Nell's caregiver will do it on Sunday morning. I may have her come earlier on Sunday, so she can take care of Nell earlier than 10:00 A.M. the time she has been coming. Normally, I have been getting her up and feeding her and she sits in her gown by the bed until Andrea comes, but in this new procedure, I can't let Nell lay in bed until 10:00 A.M. till Andrea comes for her to put Nell on the potty. If she comes an hour earlier, and I give her an extra $10.00, it is worth it to me and to Nell. This month begins a new routine of care. Can't shower Nell any more. I bathed and dressed her in bed. Now we will use the bedside potty rather than the toilet. Our bedroom looks like a nursing home residence.

9/15/2017   Friday. Yesterday I watched Shantel give Nell a sponge bath while she was sitting on the bedside commode. Then she dressed her and sat her in her chair in the living room. I fed her Ensure and orange juice with a spoonful of Mira Lax. Last night as Nell slept she turned on her right side and faced me during the night, kicking her feet. She woke me up several times kicking me with her foot or knee. This is the first time in a long time that she hasn't just laid on her back all night long in the same position.

Shantel bathed Nell in bed this morning after they (Shantel & Andrea) were aware that Nell's right knee was sore and she would not stand on it. Later in the day, she did walk on it a lot better. When I got home from golf, I got her up from the couch and walked her to her chair. She sat there till bedtime. I put her on the bedside potty and changed from her clothes to her pajamas and Depends. I cleaned her and layed her down in bed. Her eyes were a little red and teary, so I put some eye drops in them. She watched the news with me a few minutes and went to sleep. She had a down day. She was weak and listless. Her life force seemed to be weakening.

9/16/2017 Saturday. I got up this morning and made some bisquits and sausage gravy for breakfast, then Carrie came and shared a bisquit. She helped me get Nell up and dress her before she went to do her Saturday activities. Nell seemed to be alright this morning. We ate breakfast in the breakfast area. We were able to get her in the wheel chair and take her to her chair in the living room.

9/17/2017 Sunday. I got Nell up this morning about 7:30 A.M. and put her on the bedside potty. Put her robe on her and sat her in the bedside chair and fed her Ensure and orange juice with Mira Lax. Andrea, her caregiver came at 9:00 A.M. and gave her a shower. She could do it, I can't. It is too dangerous for me. Andrea told me when I returned from worship and lunch, that when Nell showered she gave evidence of her feminine issue. Later when she changed her Depends, the issue had ended. She seemed to do alright in the afternoon. She stayed awake after her afternoon nap, and stared out the window. She was not interested in the TV.

At bedtime the Lord led me to sit beside her after I put her to bed. I read Psalm 20 and read it again making it read with Nell's name and then sung the doxology & Lord's Prayer.

9/18/2017 Monday. I put Nell on the bedside potty before bedtime. I put her in bed and she slept the night through. I woke her up this morning about 7:45 A.M. and put her on the potty. The Kindred Care Hospice Aid, Kenya, came about 8:15 A.M., and we took her to the shower. We had a difficult time giving her a shower. Kenya said her orders on the I-Pad, was to give her a sponge bath rather than a shower, because she had given evidence last week to be too weak to give her a shower. I think we need to bathe her in bed from now on. The wound on her knee was bleeding and we put a new bandage on it this morning. We brought her into the living room, where I fed her Ensure for breakfast.

9/19/2017 Last night I read the 23 Psalm and played Christian hymns from Pandora on the IPad. Nell went to sleep like a child. I read Colossians chapter three to Nell last night and played Christian hymns from Pandora on my IPad. She closed her eyes, but when I got up to dress for bed, she opened her eyes and followed me around the room with her eyes

9/20/2017 Wednesday. Today, I go to senior choir rehearsal at Dauphin Way Baptist Church. The aid will come and bathe and dress Nell, then Andrea our caregiver will come and be with Nell from 10:00 A.M. until 2:00 P.M. The last few days, Nell has been about the same. She will sleep or watch TV, mostly sleep. Several nights now, I have put Nell to bed, and sat down beside her and read scripture to her. When she was growing up, her mother and aunt used to read stories to her while she went to sleep. So when I read scripture, she immediately closes her eyes just like she did, I imagine, as a little child. Last night I read Psalm 23. Then, I played some hymn singing, from Pandora on my Ipad, and let it play for some time. If I did anything unusual, she would open her eyes immediately. She has some thought processes going on that she can't express because she can't talk. She does express some thought through her body language. When I put her on her potty chair before putting her to bed it is a tough physical effort. I have to pick her up from the wheel chair and turn 180 degrees to put her on the potty chair. To lift her from the potty chair to bed is also difficult. If I have to clean her she will lean over while I clean from behind. She will put her head down, and after she is all cleaned and ready to be lifted in bed, she keeps her head down. I think, in embarrassment. It is pitiful. But, I try to make her feel comfortable and I look at her and say, "I love you." She seems to perk up a little after that. Last night when I told her I was going to read scripture to her, she opened her blue eyes wide and just stared at me. I looked right back at her and did not look away, but talked to her. I did not see any response in her eyes, but I was not going to look away, so there in those few moments, she just stared at me. After some time she looked away at something else.

9/21/2017　　　Thursday, the last day of summer. I played golf today in a Minister's golf tournament. Andrea was Nell's caregiver today. Jan, the Kindred Care Nurse came and checked Nell's vitals and all was well. Nell's finger was swollen and it was swelled around her rings. Jan said to soak her finger in warm water with some dish soap, and give her some Ibuprofen twice a day after meals to help the swelling go down. Nell's right knee is swollen. I think it is arthritis. She may have had a slight stroke also, because she cannot lift her right leg. Orders from Kindred Hospice are not to walk her into a shower, but to give her a sponge bath. She has had a good attitude the last three or four days.

9/22/17　　　Friday, the first day of Fall, and it is 4:00 A.M. I couldn't sleep, even after playing golf on Thursday. I wasn't tired after the game. But, I had an unsettled feeling, when I went to bed, and I guess while I slept, and for no reason, as far as I could think of any. Taking care of Nell –when you think of it – is not that hard. Each little task, is easy. I am getting used to her sitting on the potty chair and cleaning her. Then I put on the night gown, and pull up her "diapers." That is a little difficult because I have to stand her up and she is "wobbly." Getting her in bed is probably the hardest thing, because I have to lay her back on the bed and then move and lift her upper body on the pillow and lift her legs up on the bed, and slowly get her in a comfortable position. Getting her up in the morning and sitting her on the potty by the bed and taking her night gown off, is not that hard. I have to hold her as I move her about. Each little task in itself is not hard. During the day, she sits on her chair with her legs up and sleeps or watches TV, or just "looks" at the patio door and the view beyond. When I talk to her or feed her, or get her up from the chair to lay her down on the couch for a nap after lunch, she has no response. Nell's finger is swelled around her ring. Last night after I soaked her hand in warm, soapy water, I removed her rings from her finger because I was concerned that the circulation was being cut off. She showed no response to the procedure. All these little tasks are not hard in themselves, but for some reason, in an aggregate, they cause an unsettled feeling in my stomach. But, I am even getting used to an unsettled feeling. I just notice it once in a while, but I think it is constant. When I am busy, my mind is on something else, and I don't notice it, but when I sit, soon I realize I have an unsettled stomach, a nervous stomach, a worrisome spirit.

When I minister to Nell, I talk to her in a loving way, and realize how much I love her and "miss," her. She is losing weight as I feed her Ensure, ice cream and other things that she can drink. Her little legs and arms are pitiful. All her life, after she gave birth, she has had a little fat on her stomach. Now after all these years, that little pouch is going away. I am writing this diary, to explain to anyone who has this same experience to be encouraged, because I believe it is easier to take care of your spouse at home, rather than her being in a nursing home. I think of how they are taking care of her while I am not in sight. I realize that they don't care for her like I do at home. After I have put her in a nursing home, while I have respite care several times, now twice, that it is not good. I have a caregiver that comes in several times during the week, and an aid from Kindred Hospice who comes in each weekday morning and bathes, and dresses her. The rest of the time, it is "on" me. I would rather she be here in her own home, than in a nursing home, where I would go and minister to her there. I would rather do it here, with the help with which I am blessed. For Nell, in her condition, it couldn't be any better. And, I believe for me, this is best, also. So, I have an unsettled stomach watching her deteriorate physically, she has already deteriorated mentally, I ask myself, "So What?" Suck it up. It is another day coming, and God is there in mysterious ways. The scripture says, "Call upon me and I will answer you and show you great and mighty things, which you knowest not." One of the great and mighty things is, I am doing these tasks and watching this digression in my wife, and I am handling it as well as I am.

9/24/2017   Sunday. I got up at 4:00 A.M. this morning, because Nell kept throwing her legs around. I got some some Preparation H, later in the afternoon, and I applied it I got her ready for bed around 6:00 P.M. I went to bed around 9:30 P.M. after I was confident that Auburn would be the winner in football over Missouri. I slept until 3:30 A.M. and when I awoke, I became aware of Nell's tossing and turning and kicking her legs. She was in some discomfort so I got up and changed her Depends and applied the Preparation H. She seemed to relax and go right to sleep, so I do believe that irritation caused her unrest. One thing that got my attention was the look of peace and admiration on her face, as she looked at me when I finished applying the Prep. H. and got her Depends back on her. Later, at about 5:30 A.M. I went to check on Nell and she was sound asleep. I think that the Prep.H. gave her some soothing relief. I dressed Nell this morning after I gave her a slight sponge bath, and applied the Prep. H. Andrea cared for her today and applied the Prep. H. again after about 11:30 A.M. I applied it again after her nap, about 3:30 P.M. when I put on clean Depends.

9/25/2017   Monday 4:00 A.M. Nell was kicking me, flaying her legs, about 2:30 A.M. I tried to sleep, but finally got up, turned the light on. She was wide awake, looking at me, like – who are you? When I got her ready for bed on Sunday night, she was involved Preparation H. I put on new Depends and put her in bed. She slept until 2:30 A.M. when she started tossing her legs, so I thought she was in discomfort. When I changed her, she was soaken wet. I had to replace the absorbent blanket under her along with her Depends. I cleaned her and applied Prep. H. She appeared to relax, and just looked at me, with an appearance of gratitude. An hour later I checked to see how she was doing and she seemed to be sleeping good, so I assume the Prep. H. took away her discomfort.

9/27/2017   Tuesday. Nell slept too much today. She slept so soundly that to try to awaken her was difficult. She drank her Ensure tonight alright and she drank a little bit of a milk-shake this afternoon, about a third of a glass. When I tried to stand her up to put her in the wheel chair to take her to the bedroom to prepare her for bed, she was unable to help hold herself up on her legs and just collapsed. I could only hold her to let her down gently on the floor. I called Carrie and she sent Jeff over to help me get her in the wheel chair. At bedtime, I put her on the potty. Then I cleaned her and put her on the bed. I put on her Depends after I treated her with Preparation H. She is sleeping now or watching T.V.

I was reading my Caregiver Devotion several days ago, and the devotion was directed to the caregiver to see something unique in the patient and try to work with that. God has made a unique human being and it is the caregiver's job to talk and find out about the patient's life and try to nurture that special gift. I thought about Nell, she cannot talk, so it is hard to get her to talk, but after 63 years of marriage, I know a lot about Nell. But to try to nurture her uniqueness is difficult now. When I put her to bed last night she had a evidence of her feminine issue, when I sat her on the potty. I had to get her on the bed and roll her over so I could clean her. It took some time to clean her and then I applied the medicine on her hemorrhoids and put her Depends on her and laid her on her pillow. I attached the barrier on the bed to prevent her from falling out of bed, although she hardly moves a muscle during the night. If she is hurting or in a state of discomfort as is the case now, she kicks her legs a lot. I have to get up, change her Depends and put more Prep H. on her, then she is at peace. So after I put the Prep H. on her after the barrier is fixed, I looked at her, and instead of the "steely" stare, she had a pleasant look of admiration and peace on her face. So that was an experience to help me find her uniqueness in this stage of her life. She couldn't talk, but somewhere in her brain there was some life to where she could express her thanks by an expression in her eyes and on her face. It was interesting and a blessing to me to try to encourage that uniqueness more often. Sometimes I detect tears coming down her cheek. There is emotion there in her brain that allows that feeling to express itself in tears. This morning when I tried to awaken her, she looked like the Lord had called her home. I felt her and she was cool to the touch. I could not read a pulse right away, but finally I found a pulse. I was pleased and disappointed at the same time. I have mentioned my mixed feelings about her living before, and the stress of wanting her to live, and the emotion that comes over me when I find out she has not died. I know it is just a matter of time, and I am blessed to be healthy enough to care for her until God calls her home, but if He wants to call me to his side first, then so be it. There is a purpose in all this that is a mystery. It tries my faith and I pray for increased faith. God has honored that prayer. When I finish my devotion in the morning and prayer, I close with the Lord's Prayer and sing the Doxology. It starts out: "Praise God from whom all blessings flow."

9/28/2017   Thursday. Last night I lifted Nell up from her chair in the living room, to put her in the wheel chair to take her to the bedroom and get her in bed, and she would not help me with her legs, and I found myself holding all the weight and all I could do was to let her down on the floor easy. I could not get her back on the easy chair. I made her comfortable on the floor and called for help to lift her into the wheel chair. Jeff came and helped me. I got her in bed and we slept through the night. This morning Shantel bathed Nell and dressed her. She brought her into the living room and seated her in her easy chair. Since that time, Nell has been sleeping. She slept during my feeding her Ensure. I had to shake her head slightly to get her to sip on the straw to drink all of the Ensure. I have been so concerned, I called Jan the Nurse for Kindred Care Hospice to talk to her about my concern. Jan said it was a stage Nell is going through. She told me that she probably has forgotten how to walk. She said she will soon forget how to suck on the straw to get her sustenance. We will have to pick her up to put her in the wheel chair. She cannot walk to any degree. She has forgotten how to put one step to the next, especially when she has a pain in her right leg. I am concerned that Friday when I play golf that she might expire. Nurse Jan said that her death is not imminent, could be but not probable. She said for me to keep up my schedule as planned.

9/30/2017 Saturday. Last night when I put Nell to bed and put on clean dry Depends, I forgot to put barrier ointment on her seat and apply Prep. H. About 1:00 A.M. on Saturday, Nell was fighting in bed and I remembered I did not put the barrier ointment on her seat, nor the Prep. H. so I thought she was in discomfort. So I got up and turned the bedside light on. She was wide awake, and she looked at me with a frightened look. It was such a fear on her face it scared me to think that she thought that it was an intruder. I began to talk to her and she then relaxed. I took off the wet Depends and cleaned her, applied the barrier ointment, and Prep. H. Before I put on the clean, dry Depends, she went to sleep. I turned her on her side, because she had a slight rash on her back. She slept soundly the rest of the night. I looked in at her about 7:30 A.M. and she was sleeping. I felt real good about helping her through the night. I know she was uncomfortable in the night, and changing her was the right thing to do. She can't complain, and the only sign of discomfort she may have that I can detect is her moving around with her legs and hip area. I believe the reason she was moving around was discomfort. That is why she went to sleep and slept from about 2:00 A.M. until about 7:30 A.M. I stayed up after I got up to tend to her around 2:00 A.M., and stayed up and went back to bed about 4:00 A.M. and slept until 6:30 A.M. I made myself some breakfast and after I cleaned, dressed Nell and fed her I went out into the yard and used my weed eater .

I feel good today. I think it was because in the middle of the night I ministered to Nell to ease her discomfort and that made me feel good in the morning. I pray every morning to do my best, and ask God to show me if I have not done my best for Nell and for me to confess my sin of disregard in some manner if I am not taking good care of Nell. I think God has infused me with His Spirit for my faithfulness to carry out my part of the prayer to do my best, even in discerning Nell's discomfort and remembering that I did not put the barrier ointment on her seat, and the Prep. H. which relieves the itching and burning. God has been so faithful to me when I am obedient to his voice and urging. How could I do otherwise, to the life time partner in bringing a wonderful family into being and doing all she could all her life to be a wonderful, loving mother and wife. Every time I think I can't hold her up, and it puts great strain on my back, to lift her to bed, or to her potty or to the wheel chair or into her chair, I think, "I need to put her in a nursing home before I am "down" myself. Then I think, a night like last night, the nursing home nurses would let her be in discomfort all night and probably would not change her until about 9:00 or 10:00 A.M. when they got around to it. Nell could not complain because she cannot talk. So she would have laid in bed all night in discomfort. But I am sleeping next to her and discern her need, and take care of the discomfort.

10/1/2017   Sunday. For several months, a person I regarded as a good friend and counselor to our family on the matter of Nell's Alzheimer disease, has been avoiding me when I see her. I have prayed over the reason, and I am sure it is something I have done or said that may have influenced this behavior. I saw her husband this morning and said to him that I believe his wife, whom I respect greatly for her help in the beginning of Nell's disease, has been avoiding me when I see her. I told him that if I have caused her any hurt, I want to apologize. Her husband said that he knew of nothing. I think he was covering for her. But I shall continue to pray that she would reestablish our relationship, for I need her friendship at a time like this with Nell, in the latter stages of Alzheimer's. I don't know what to do, for I do not want to force myself on her if she feels some stress in our meeting or in our relationship. God will work this out.

Nell has been doing well today. Andrea took care of her well, and it is soon the time for me to feed her Ensure for the evening and get her ready for bed.

10/2/2017 Now into October and Nell is mostly bedridden, because of the lack of strength in her legs. Kindred Care hospice aid Shantel is bathing Nell and dressing Nell in bed now during weekday mornings. Then she puts her in wheel chair and moves her to her living room Jerry chair. I can move her from bed to potty, or potty to bed. I can move her from potty to wheel chair and to wheel chair to potty. I can move her from wheel chair to easy chair or to couch, or couch and easy chair to wheel chair. All this moving from one place to another I can do, but with very little use of her legs. She has not been out of the house now for about a month. It is difficult and unsafe for me to get her in and out of the car to wheel chair or back into the car from wheel chair. When I am pushing her in the wheel chair she scoots down and I have a difficult time getting her back into the wheel chair. So that is also unsafe. If I had a person accompany me, I could take her out, but she doesn't seem to comprehend anything, and mostly sleeps anyway. Maybe the only time to take her out would be to the doctor, to get her nails done, or to the hair solon to cut her hair, but I would need help.

Today, Kenya has come to bathe her in bed and dress her. She will put her in the wheel chair and bring her into the living room and put her into the Jerry chair, and I will feed her. After that, she will watch TV, where she sleeps mostly after she eats. I will clean the ceramic floors today.

When I get up in the morning, my stomach seems to be upset, or an anxious feeling. In past days I would have thought it was because of anxiety over all the work to get Nell ready for the day. I would shower her and dress and feed her. That became a burden, as I did it day after day, and when I would get up, I was full of stress for what was immediately ahead of me for the day.

But now Kindred Care Aids come and do all that. The aid this morning (Kenya) even made the bed. I don't have anxiety over taking care of Nell, but I think I have anxiety over her physical condition and a worry, that she is going to die soon, but how soon, that is the worry. Will it be in the night while I am beside her, or will it be after I get up in the morning and return to get her up and find that the Lord has called her home. On the one hand I believe I will be relieved, and on the other great sorrow. I know that I will miss her presence greatly, even though she doesn't seem to respond or show any evidence of recognizing me or any one for that matter.

10/5/2017   Thursday. I hope Nell has not gone to another stage in her illness today. This afternoon, she would just drink a few drinks of her Ensure, and later I tried to mix the Ensure with a glass of milkshake. She did drink that, however slowly and with some resistance. This afternoon, Pat the social worker came by and checked Nell out to evaluate her. She comes once a month, and commented that Nell has declined quite a bit since the last time she was here.

10/7/2017   Saturday. This is the one day of the week, I don't have an aid or caregiver to bathe and dress Nell. Last night I did not transfer Nell from her Jerry chair to the wheel chair properly and she slipped off the wheel chair and all I could do was to let her down on the floor gently. I put a pillow under her head and laid her there until I could get help. After about 30 minutes, Jeff was able to come and help me lift her in to the wheel chair. I was able to get her on the potty, and dress her for bed. Normally, she would sit on the potty before I put her to bed. But with all the exertion in getting her up from the floor and on to the wheel chair, she had an accident. I had a tedious job getting her clean, applying ointment and Prep. H., and putting on her Depends. She went right to sleep after she was prepared for bed. However, in the early morning, she kicked her legs a lot and this movement awoke me. I could not get back to sleep , so I finally got up. It is 2:00 A.M. I don't know if she is in some discomfort, she can't tell me. I don't know what to do. I will go to check on her after some time and see if she is asleep, and if not I will put the lights on and try to talk to her and see if I can discern any pain. And if she seems to be in pain I will give her two Ibuprofin pills.

10/8/2017   Sunday. We did not have church services today due to Hurricane Nate. Andrea did not come to sit with Nell. I bathed Nell in bed and dressed her mostly in bed. I put her in the wheel chair and pushed her in her Jerry chair to the living room and fed her. She drank her Ensure, both at breakfast and lunch. She slept most of the time since I put her there after I got her up. There is a lot of declining: she has declined in bathing, first in the bathtub, to shower and now bathing in bed. Also, she is declining in dressing. I used to dress her after a bath, and she would assist. Then I could not bathe her anymore so I showered her. Then I would dress her with some ease. That got progressively more dangerous, so we started bathing her in bed, and then dressing her in bed. She declined in her eating habits. She began a decline in eating when I would help direct her spoon or fork to her mouth, or help get food on the utinsel, and help her get it to her mouth. Then it got to where I would have to feed her. After awhile, she would not eat solid food, and I resorted to just giving her Ensure. Now the Ensure has been going on for about six months. The whole declining process has taken about a year. She used to stay awake quite a bit and I could take her in the car, then put her in a wheel chair and she would sit at the restaurant table while I ate. I would feed her Ensure. Now, for the last month, I have not been able to get her in the car and then into the wheel chair to take her with me, so I have not taken her out of the house for at least six weeks now. Now she sleeps mostly, and starting Saturday, she has mostly slept or watched TV with her mouth open. Today, she has slept since she got up and it is now 2:00 PM. Her mouth is open, and she looks like she is deceased. I can wake her, but her eyes are not awake. When I quit trying to keep her awake, she just goes back to sleep. She can't live much longer with no stimulation, just sleeping. It is heartbreaking to see her like this. Although, she did drink her Ensure at lunch, even while appearing to be asleep.

10/9/2017   Monday. Today, I had Andrea come to sit with Nell because she did not come on Sunday, due to the Church being closed because of hurricane Nate. I wanted to make sure she draws a salary by caregiving for Nell at least three days a week. Nell is more alert today and she is eating better today. Tonight I will go to Nell's Murphy H.S. alumni dinner in place of Nell. Calvin will come and stay with her while I am absent. I will put her to bed when I return. Normally I get her to bed about 7:00 P.M.. but tonight it will be closer to 8:00 P.M. Nell seemed to be alert and watched TV at times today.

10/11/2017   I am unable to describe my feelings as Nell declines. It is worse as I awaken. I feel nervous in the stomach and feel weak, even, in my legs, but that description does not adequately explain the feeling. Sometimes when she drops her chin with her mouth wide open and has a dark penetrating stare in her eyes it frightens me.

10/12/2017   Thursday. I lost several days of entry in my diary. I posted some earlier things about the caregiver. I have been having an upset stomach, or nervous stomach after I awaken in the morning. This morning I almost threw up. I think it is because I live minute by minute thinking that Nell has died. I lay beside her at night and put my arm around her and she feels cold. I check her pulse and she has a heartbeat. When she sits in her chair during the day and falls asleep, she looks like she has died, and when I go to her and check to see, she is still living. I live minute by minute thinking Nell has died. I can't help thinking that Alzheimer's has a death grip on me as well as Nell. It is as if death is saying, "I will draw you to death with this disease. I will linger and delay my coming to

Nell and cause you both to go the way of all men, together." I say to myself, that this may be so, but meanwhile, I will do all I can to keep Nell as well as I can. I will be as if I told death, "I know your game." Just by admitting what is on my mind, what is causing my upset stomach, relieves my anxiety. It seems I am in a battle with death the same as Nell. The disease is taking it's hourly toll on Nell, and it tries to take its toll on me also, but I will resist and fight Alzheimer's death threat on me. I can outlast death's threat on me and let it know that I know it's game. I will walk alongside it's threat and be with Nell as best as I can, and see things clearly. God will take Nell when it's His hour of choosing, and God will choose me also, in His hour of choosing and for me it will have little to do with Alzheimer's disease.

I think as the days drag on my life is mostly in caregiving. I don't want to sound begrudging, but, it is life that is appointed unto me by the turn of events that I dress and undress, then feed, and clean, and this is all done around Nell's sleeping. She is sleeping in bed, sleeping in her Jerry chair or sleeping on the couch. I have to change her from one sleeping position to another during the day. That is her life now; getting up from bed to sleep and eat. What a turn of events that her life has just come to that. But Alzheimer's is the controlling factor.

10/13/2017   I get up in the morning feeling nauseous at times not knowing why, not having any definite reason, but I am sure it is emotional or mental. After I take a shower, dress and walk, I feel better. Today, I have a time to get away from caregiving for several hours while I play golf. The diversion and friends help me feel better

10/14/2017   Saturday. Nell started her feminine issue again Thursday. Last night, (Friday) I got her ready for bed and she did not have evidence since I changed her Depends after her nap, so hopefully, it has ended. It is 6:00 A.M., I have been up since 3:30 A.M. I could not sleep after I got up at 2:00

A.M. to go to the bathroom, so I got up and read, had my devotion, got breakfast ready. Then at 5:00 A.M. I laid down in my chair and tried to sleep, which I did in a kind of catnap, and finally got up from the chair at 6:00 P.M. It came to my mind while catnapping, that Nell is going to be healed and we will be as she was before she got Alzheimer's disease. I thought this may be like a cold, or flu or cancer even. But no! This is not a "get well" kind of disease. This is a permanent declining and terminal illness. Makes me depressed to think that all the good times in semi-retirement we were having, will never be returning. We will not be picking up where we left off, when Nell got Alzheimer's. It is not like a cold. Life as we knew it will not be returning. In essence, our lives are over. Nell is 81 years of age, and I am 87. This is how lives end, how they terminate, by illness, by cancer, by heart attack, and some by Alzheimer's. Nell was alert mostly today. She watched football with me all day up through Alabama's game which ended about 10:00 PM. The only time she slept was when I laid her down for her nap in the afternoon.

10/15/2017   Sunday, I awakened Nell and fed her in bed this morning. Andrea will be here at 9:30 A.M., to bathe her and dress her. She seems alert this morning as she did all day Saturday. We watched football all day and into the evening when the Alabama/Arkansas game ended about 10:00 P.M. The only time she slept was when I laid her down for a nap around noon until 2:00 P.M. She slept well last night. I am not needing to apply Preparation H.

10/16/2017 Monday. Last night Carrie called me to discuss buying a travel trailer and parking it next to her house, and my staying there after Nell dies, and I had my phone on speaker and Nell heard this. I immediately turned off the speaker and discussed this subject quietly on the phone with Carrie. Later, as we watched TV together, I noticed a tear on her cheek. I looked at her closely and she was weeping, and her chin was dropped and quivering. I asked her if she was hurting. She just looked at me with this hurt look. I think she overheard our conversation, and was able to comprehend the conversation. When I put her to bed, I read scripture and played some Christian hymns on my I-pad. She went to sleep, and slept soundly through the night. I put my arm around her and held her hand when I got in bed, hoping that I could comfort her, if indeed she did comprehend our conversation. When I put her to bed last night she had her feminine issue again like she was having a menstrual period. She was involved in this for a couple days, then stopped for several days, and began again during the afternoon. This morning, (Monday) the Kindred Care Aid said she was alright. She has been sleeping mostly this morning. It is now 11:00 A.M.

10/17/2017   I hurt real bad this morning to think God will let Nell linger in this way in life and not take her or not heal her.

10/18/2017   Wednesday. It hurts my heart to see Nell, previously so active in life, now so pitiful. She can't do anything except drink Ensure and then go to the potty. Yesterday, when she was not sleeping, she just stared. I don't know if she is in pain, cold or hot. She can't speak, she can't smile or frown. She mostly just stares. I can't understand why God allows her to linger in this distressful condition for her and for her loved ones and friends. Why doesn't God heal her, or take her to be with him? He is a loving God, but I can't see the love expressed in allowing her to go on like this. What good is this for her, for me and the children? They don't like to remember her in this manner. They want to have the good memories. Well, today again, we will take this situation from the hand of God, and one day see the good of it, even though we can't understand it now. We have to trust, in so many words from God, that we cannot understand. Words like "all things work together for good to those who love God," and also verses like John 14, 12, 13, where Jesus says that "those who believe in Him will do the works that He does, but greater works will we do because

He will go to the Father. Whatsoever you ask of God it shall be done so that the Father will be glorified in the son. If you ask anything in my name, it shall be done." I have asked for healing for Nell and for mercy. What healing has come? What mercy that I am looking to and understand has come? I am grateful to God that I have been blessed with health to take care of Nell.

10/20/2017   Friday. Yesterday, I played in a golf tournament, and Andrea stayed with Nell. Kim and Pat came down from Huntsville. They had things to do and we all got home about 2:00 P.M. Thursday evening Kim fixed a meal and all the Mobile family was here and we ate on the patio. I wheeled Nell out on the patio in her Jerry Chair. I don't know if she was aware of the get together or not, but at least she was with us. Kim and Carrie divided up a lot of Nell's clothes she could not wear. Kim is going to take what they could not use, and put the clothes in a second hand clothes store, or consignment store. Nell did alright in the crowd of people and seemed to be glad to be in bed. Today, now, she appears to be quite sluggish. She has no energy, her eyes are sleepy looking, and her mouth is agape. She doesn't look good. My heart is hurt with her appearance. I fed her the noon Ensure and laid her down on the couch for a nap.

10/21/2017   Barely Saturday (12:30 A.M.) I went to bed last night the same time when I put Nell to bed at 6:30 P.M. I watched the news, then watched the beginning of a movie and was so sleepy by 8:00 P.M. I turned the movie off and went to sleep. I woke up at 12:00 A.M. wide awake. Nell was kicking her legs and that caused me to stay awake also, so I decided to get up. Yesterday (Friday), Nell had a good day, except sluggish, and drowsy all day. When I put her to bed last night it was a struggle. It takes a lot of back lifting. The last few days I have been feeling some pain in my back which has been a worry. I think if my back gets more painful, I will have to put Nell in a nursing home. I will talk to Jan, the nurse from Kindred

Care Hospice to find out if there is any other alternative for help to keep her at home. I told Nell last night when I was putting her to bed that if my back is not able to move her during the day and put her to bed at night I might have to put her in a nursing home. She was looking at me, and her eyes got rounder and alert as if to say, "No, don't do that." She is so helpless.

I got Nell up this morning and dressed her. I took her into the living room to transfer her from the wheel chair to the Jerry chair and as I was lifting her from the wheel chair she fell on the floor. I was able to catch her enough to let her down gently and hold her head up so she would not hit her head. She pulled me down with her. I got up and put a pillow under her head. Calvin was able to come and help me get her into the Jerry chair. I fed her and since then she has been sleeping. It is now 10:30 A.M.

10/22/2017   Sunday. Yesterday Nell was unusually groggy. Her eyes would verily open. In the evening while preparing for bed, she began to be more alert. During the night she tried to cuddle with me by throwing her legs across my body and holding my hand. When I tried to change positions and needed my hand, she would just grip my hand tightly. This morning she was awake when I got up about 5:00 A.M. But later went back to sleep and woke up again about 8:00 A.M. and I fed her in bed. I will let Andrea bathe and dress her. She will bring her to the living room and place her in the Jerry chair.

Andrea said that Nell did good while I went to church and dinner after worship services. When I got home Nell was laying down for a nap. I let her sleep until 4:00 P.M. I got her up and put her in the Jerry Chair. She mostly slept after that until she somewhat opened her eyes and watched a movie until I put her to bed around 6:15 P.M. Her legs are getting weaker and it is becoming quite difficult to get her from the Jerry chair to the wheel chair and from the wheel chair to the potty, and from the potty to bed. If she can help a little with any strength she has in her legs I can do all that. But when her legs give way I have to carry her over the potty. And when they give way when I lift her from the potty, I have to have her over the bed to sit her on the edge of the bed. If her legs give way between the wheel chair and potty, or the potty to the bed, she will collapse on the floor, and I will have to make her comfortable until I can get help to lift her up from the floor. Tonight, she had tears in her eyes when I put her to bed. I think she has some emotional response when I have to clean her after her potty and when I get her in bed to make sure she is clean to put on her Depends. She just looks at me and tears are in her eyes. Not so much as they would run down her cheeks, but just enough to be on her cheeks.

10/24/2017   Tuesday . Nell was alert yesterday, but this morning about 10:30 A.M., she is very sleepy, groggy eyes when open. She just wants to sleep. She seemed to sleep well last night.

I have written in my diary that death not only attacks the Alzheimer's victim, but also the spouse caregiver. A minister friend of mine told me that his mother had Alzheimer's and is still living after 20 years with the disease. He said he watched his father go down and finally die being his wife's caregiver. I thought about that and I want to be a good caregiver for Nell, but also be a good caregiver for me. But if I die during my caregiving efforts to be a good caregiver, then I will be obedient to this responsibility unto death. I am 87 and will die any time. I could die working in the yard, eating in a restaurant, or playing golf. We will all die, but when and where and under what physical condition? We don't know, but we can be faithful to the responsibility we have been assigned and standing tall in the midst of it when God calls us to be with Him. The important thing is to be ready to meet God. I am confident of my life with God on the basis of my faith in Jesus Christ through his grace and mercy.

10/25/2017   Nell has been involved with her feminine issue again now for three days. It seems to be more evident, in the evening, when I change her Depends to put her to bed.

10/26/2017   Thursday. I have not entered any notes the last few days because Nell's condition has been pretty level in her wellbeing and in my caregiving status. The only thing that is continuing is her feminine issue. It was fairly heavy last night. The Kindred Care Hospice nurse will be here today to make her weekly check up. She came and said all went well, her vital signs were good.

10/27/2017   Friday. The only comment today is that there is no evidence of her issue. I slept last night with a troubled spirit, mixed up and troubled dreams, got up about 5:30 AM. showered and shaved, determined with God's help, to change my attitude from troubled to one of joy and thanksgiving.

10/28/2017   Saturday. I talked to Nurse Jan from Kindred Care Hospice Thursday to have a hospital bed sent to our house on Tuesday, Nov. 2. It will be easier to raise the bed and lower it; also to raise her head to feed Nell rather than put pillows under her head to feed her. It is back straining to do that and uncomfortable for Nell. Carrie was talking to a Nurse, named Kim at her Bible study on Thursday night about our situation and condition of Nell. She called Kindred Care with my permission, and the results were that Nell will begin oxygen when they bring the bed. Also, the nurse from Kindred Care will also begin visiting Nell three times a week rather than just the one visit on Thursday.

4:00 A.M. on Saturday. I woke up about 3:15 A.M. and felt Nell, and found her to be soaken wet from perspiration. I got up and changed her top and the pad under her which was soaken also. I woke her up, of course, in all of the turning and changing. She just looked at me with affectionate eyes as if to say, "Thank you." When I finished she went right back to sleep.

Calvin came over to my house on Saturday and helped me arrange the bedroom furniture to accommodate a hospital bed, which will be delivered on Tuesday. Also on Tuesday, Direct TV will come and change the TV to another wall.

10/29/2017   Sunday. Last night was the first night for us to sleep in the bedroom with the new arrangement of furniture. Nell seemed to be quite normal in getting ready for bed; the potty routine was different, getting her in bed on a different side, the putting on of the Depends. This morning she had kicked off all the covers and was sleeping soundly. I put the covers back over her and it did not appear to disturb her.

10/30/17   Monday. Everything is ready in our bedroom for a hospital bed, and oxygen to be delivered and set up tomorrow, Tuesday. Hopefully this will make care for Nell easier on the caregiver and oxygen to help Nell to be more alert.

10/31/2017   Tuesday. Yesterday was my son's 62nd birthday. One week ago was Nell's and my 63rd Wedding anniversary. Today, I just had a hospital bed delivered and placed in our bedroom. Tonight will be the first time since Nell and I were married that we slept in separate beds. 63 years we have slept together, and tonight we will sleep in separate beds. For several years now, I have had to readjust my caregiving methods according to Nell's physical abilities to function. When she could not feed herself, then to when she could not eat solid food, and now she can just drink Ensure with a straw or sip it, but no solid food, and no ability to feed herself the Ensure. Then there was the time where she could no longer bathe in the bathtub and I had to help her shower. Then there was a time when she was unable to dress herself, and I had to dress her. There was a time where she accidentally wet herself. I began to put on pull up Depends. Then later after awhile, I had to begin putting on the regular diaper Depends. There was a time when she would get into bed with my careful watching. Then it came to where I would have to help her get in bed. Then there came the time that I would have to get her in bed with some help from her. There came the time when she was unable to dress herself for bed. When she was unable to dress herself for bed, I would have to put on pull up Depends and put on the night clothes and put her in bed. Now I have to put her on the chair potty, then clean her, and put on the regular Depends while she is in bed. I have to apply some protective cream and Depends and pull her gown down and cover her with the bed covers, and turn off the light. I remember when I used to put her on the toilet and she would clean herself, and now when she goes to the chair potty, I have to clean her. There will be a time when she will be unable to sit on the chair potty, and I will have to change her Depends in the bed and clean her. Gradually these different stages come in the life of the caregiver. I never thought I would be able to clean her after she sat on the toilet. But gradually, I believe, because I have been cleaning her in various stages, now, I could clean her in bed and put on her Depends in bed.

10/31/2017　　　Wednesday. I reflect back over Nell's first night in the hospital bed. She kept her eyes on me when I put her to bed and kept them on me as, later, when I went to bed. Usually she would go to sleep, but she stayed awake probably because no TV (not hooked up on other wall yet). It was Halloween and great grandchildren and Carrie and Calvin and grand daughter Kim came to visit her. She seemed perplexed in her countenance. She slept well and snored at times. She kicked all the covers off of her by 11:00 PM, but did not kick them off after that. I felt alone and hurt in my feelings to put her in a hospital bed, to be separate in bed from me after 63 years. I wonder if I am doing right by having her sleep separate in a hospital bed. I think it gave her some security and comfort to touch me during the night. The hospital bed makes it easier for the caregiver and for me to care for her, because I can raise and lower the bed while I put her to bed, and just raise the head to give the Ensure and orange juice for breakfast prior to the Kindred Care Hospice Aid bathing her and dressing her in the hospital bed. It all worked out well this morning and I brought her into the living room in the Jerry chair. I don't use the wheel chair any more. Andrea will be here at 10:00 A.M. for me to go to senior choir rehearsal and lunch with Carlton Berry.

11/2/2017   I tried to put the oxygen on Nell last night, but it made a noise that was disturbing. There was a motor sound plus the girgling of the water. She would not sleep until I shut it off. I include myself in that also. She was sleeping soundly when I got up this morning about 5:30 AM.

11/3/2017   Friday. Things have been in a regular manner these last few days. The only new thing is the sleeping arrangement. Nell has been sleeping in her hospital bed. I had the TV put on the wall where she could watch TV when she went to sleep, and when she wakes up in the morning waiting for the Kindred Aid to come bathe and dress her. This morning a substitute aid was filling in for Shantel, and at 9:00 A.M. she was still not here so I cleaned Nell and dressed her. About 11:00 A.M. the substitute aid called to say she was on the way to our house to bathe and dress Nell, and I told her that I already had her dressed. I did not need her at that hour. Nell slept well last night. When I got up at night I checked to see if she was covered and comfortable. She looked like she was dead. I was going to check her pulse, and as I did she moved, so I got back into bed. It was about 1:30 A.M. and I couldn't go back to sleep. I got up and went back to bed about 4:00 A.M. and slept till 6:30 A.M. Jan, Kindred Hospice nurse came while I was dressing Nell, and she checked her vitals. All her vitals were in good shape.

I was up early in the morning and as I usually do, I did my devotions and prayed at that hour. I made a covenant with God and Nell back in the beginning of my caregiving journey and I pray that prayer each morning during my devotions. I will insert it at this place in my journal, even though It began some time in the past.

3/2017 My daily covenant began:

Nell has Alzheimer's and God, You have placed her in my care these many years (since 1954; 63 years). We have walked side by side along our pilgrimage on this earth for all these years. First of all I ask for Nell's healing of this disease. It is a mystery why my prayers and the prayer of others have not brought healing. Increase my faith and be merciful and not let Nell suffer if physical healing is not in your plans for Nell. It is a small thing for me to stay by her side during this disease. I don't want to side step the trouble that has come to us through Nell's Alzheimer's disease in order to cope or to make it easier for me to care for her. Help me live in the power of the cross so that I would not ignore and look the other way regarding the problems of the daily, even hourly needs of Nell, in order to cope better even though it hurts me to see her physical discomfort and helplessness. God help me so I would not drift into a mental place where I resign myself to what is said to be on Nell's part, a state of no conscious awareness due to the disease, and not do my best for her. My prayer and need is for Your presence dear God to help me minister to Nell's needs in the trouble she is in so I can make her last hours on earth an easy exit and a joyful entrance into Your presence the hour of Your choosing. And, after I put her in bed each night let me look back over the day and if I have not done my best then forgive me for my negligence. Let me sense Your presence and help to be counted a faithful husband and caregiver. Help me to love as You loved. Let my obedience be unto death even as Yours was. And, if You take me from this earthly existence before Nell, I don't want it thought that I shirked my duty in any way to care for Nell in my last days while it was possible for me to be a faithful caregiver, nor to be embarrassed when I stand before You, God. I just ask You God to increase my faith and be merciful to Nell and to me, mentally, physically and financially. All this I ask in the name of our Lord Jesus Christ.

In the prayer of the early Christian father, John Baillie: Oh Thou whose love to man was proven in the passion and death of Jesus Christ our Lord, let the power of His cross be with me today. Let me love as You loved. Let my obedience be unto death. In leaning upon Your cross let me not refuse my own; yet in bearing mine, let me bear it by Your strength.

In worship today, a Christian song reminded me that troubles come to all and reveal our love for God, and give us an opportunity to grow stronger. We may decide to grow stronger. We may become faithless because of trouble. We may turn away from God. God is aware of our trouble, and in some cases, He may cause it in order to glorify Himself through trouble like He did to Job. And He may do it as He did to Jesus Christ in the crucifixion. Jesus said "Call upon me and I will show you great and wonderful things which you knowest not. I am Nell's chief caregiver. Most days the only regular person I see is the Kindred Care Hospice aid who gives Nell a bath and dresses her, or the nurse to check Nell out, or the caregiver who comes to give me some relief in caring for Nell. I get lonely for family members to come share my hurt for Nell, but I know they are busy in their lives and family, and I do not want to put guilt on them or to judge them in the time they give to see their mother or grandmother. In my eyes whatever time is given to Nell, by family, to me probably, is not enough.

11/5/2017   Sunday. Last night when I put Nell to bed, she had watery eyes and her eyes were slightly closed, barely able to see out of them. I called the nurse Jan and told her that Nell's eyes did not look good. I told her I was going to take her to Urgent Care after worship today. She suggested I put a warm compress over her eyes. So, I put warm compresses over her eyes every 15 minutes for several hours. This morning they look much better. I didn't know what was wrong with her eyes last night. This is Sunday night and her eyes look better. I did not take her to Urgent Care. If her eyes are not healthy looking Monday, I may call the Hospice doctor and have him send a prescription for me to apply to her eyes.

11/6/2017   Monday. Nell had a different Kindred Hospice Aid this morning, named Toni. She was here at 7:15 A.M. I am not used to going back on regular time, from daylight savings time, but this earlier time is best for us.

11/7/2017   I pray that you would help our family to visit with her Nannie Whitfield while she is still alive. I know it is hard, to see Nannie like this but it is part of life. We also, will get to that stage in life possibly and will want our loved one's to visit us and speak love into our eyes and heart. Nell has a growth on her cheek that does not heal. I have an appointment with a dermatologist on Wednesday (11-8) to see if it is cancerous. If it is cancerous, then to treat it. Her eyes have been watering and red. Maybe the dermatologist can tell me if it is Pinkeye. If so, I can get Kindred Hospice to order a prescription.

11/8/2017   Wednesday. It is 3:30 A.M. in the morning. I woke up at 2:30 A.M. after getting in bed about 8:30 P.M. Tuesday night. I watched TV for about a half of an hour, turned the lights out and was asleep. I went with a group of men from Dauphin Way Baptist Church to play golf at Cambrian Ridge Golf Course in Greenville, Alabama. Lynn Sigouin and Linda Martin came and stayed with Nell from 8:00 A.M. until 3:00 P.M. Andrea came to stay with Nell and put her to bed about 6:30 P.M. I got home from playing golf at 7:15 P.M. Andrea did a good job of putting Nell to bed and had the oxygen on her and Nell was sound asleep when I got home. When I checked her oxygen mask, it was off to the side.

When I got up this morning Wednesday, about 2:30 A.M. it was off on the side of her cheek, again. Now, today at 1:30 P.M. I am taking Nell to the dermatologist to have a cancer treated that is located on her left cheek.

11/9/2017   Thursday. I took Nell to Dr. Scott Freeman, dermatologist, yesterday, and he cut the whole area around the skin cancer, and told me to bring her back in a year. I am sure he took enough of the area that he got all the cancer. He said not to be concerned. The cut was about the size of a dime. She winced when he gave her several shots around the area in order to remove the cancer without pain. The doctor also looked at her eyes which have been watering and were a little red around the eyelids. He said she had an eye infection and prescribed a medicine to put in her eyes twice a day. It was about 2:00 P.M. when I left the doctor's office. I called the receptionist at Dauphin Way Baptist Church to have any of the staff who wanted to, to come out to the drive-through cover and say hello to Nell. She hadn't been to church for eight months or thereabouts. They all loved Nell, and when they came and greeted her, she was so attentive and alert, looking at the women with a pleasant look on her face. They all spoke to her and I am sure it gave them and Nell a good feeling. Yesterday in riding in the car going to and returning from the doctor and church visit Nell seemed to ride somewhat alert. She did as good as she did six months ago. Although it was harder getting her in and out of the car.

11/10/2017   Nell slept on her back with the oxygen in her nose, and she appears not to have moved during the night. I checked her this morning thinking maybe she had left her body and was gone to glory. When I leaned over her she opened her eyes and looked at me momentarily and closed them in sleep again.

11/11/2017   Our granddaughter, Stacey, was having a baby shower today. I felt led through God's Spirit that to leave Nell with the caregiver and I go to Stacey's baby shower would not be right for me. Nell could travel alright but it seems to me that in bringing Nell to the shower might cause some discomfort in the gathering by her hurtful appearance.

11/17/2017   Friday. It has been a few days since I have commented on Nell's condition and activities. The last several nights, Nell has slept so soundly that several times during the night when I got up, I thought the Lord had called her to her heavenly home. She has had a slight eye infection in her left eye. I have been putting drops in both her eyes and the drops seem to be killing the infection. This morning when I got her up, and took the sheets down as I was feeding her, I noticed some blood deep in her belly button. The nurse looked at it when she came today and said it was not draining and was no cause for worry. I was concerned because it had to come from somewhere that it shouldn't. I will keep an eye on this and if it gets worse, I will consult our family doctor.

Last night, my granddaughter Kim Coleman and daughter, Carrie came for a visit. It was of the hour that I put Nell to bed. She was sitting on the potty when they came to see her. After they talked with her for a few minutes, Kim put her cheek next to Nell's lips and Nell kissed Kim on her cheek. Then Carrie put her cheek up to Nell's lips and Nell puckered up her lips and kissed Carrie on her cheek. I was astonished!

11/18/2017   Saturday. This morning as I was walking in the neighborhood for my regular walk, right after sunrise (6:20 A.M.), it came to my mind as I was praying for mercy for Nell. Healing or mercy. Then it came to me that God is being merciful in one way and that is keeping me healthy. I am doing all I can to stay healthy, but all that I try to do to keep healthy that would be nothing without God's grace to see that physically and mentally, I continue to stay healthy.

11/19/2017   For the last several months at this time Nell began to bleed as if she was having a regular menstrual period. I am hoping it doesn't happen anymore.

11/21/2017   Tuesday. Yesterday, I took Nell to Dr. Free-land, Dermatologist to have him "clean up" the cancer on her cheek. The nurse called and said I needed to bring her back, although originally he said "come back in a year." Evidently tests showed he needed to do some more work to make sure all the cancer was gone. He deadend the area with shots and then lasered the area to make sure he got all the cancer. Nell was quiet and did not wince when he put the shot in her cheek to deaden the area. I was sorry for the whole event. Getting her into the car and out of the car and into the surgery room to have the cancer removed. Then home and moving her into her Jerry chair. Then to put Nell to bed, with all that is required in that was a tired day for Nell. First the potty, then cleaning her, then putting on a barrier cream, then treating her hem-morroids. Then putting on her wrap around Depends is a pro-cess. I like the hospital bed, because I can lower the bed to put her on it from the potty. I can raise it to make it easier on my back in getting her cleaned and dressed to be ready for sleep. Then I attach the oxygen, and put drops into her eyes. When I turn out the lights she sometimes watches TV, until she goes to sleep. Last night she went right to sleep.

I thought last night when I put the drops into her eyes look-ing into her eyes prior to the drops was an endearing look. She was looking at me with her big blue eyes and there was a look of thanks for all you do. It was a bonding moment for her and me. Every night I put her to bed, and do my best to be loving and kind, undressing and putting on her pajamas to make her comfortable. I think, that if she was in a nursing home, the aid would not treat her the way I do. That bonding would be missed, each night during this delicate time dealing with some personal things in getting her ready to sleep for the night. (In editing this, as I look back on treating the cancer, I would not have done it, if I had an idea that the end of her life was so near. You never know). Putting Nell to bed at night is a bonding experience. It opens my heart to God's love which I can extend to Nell.

11/22/2017   Wednesday. 3:00 PM I layed Nell down for her nap on the hospital bed in our bedroom, instead of on the couch in the living room. The reason for the change was Britanie (Granddaughter from Huntsville) was bringing my lunch to me and I did not want then to disturb her while she was sleeping. When I put her on her hospital bed, I closed the bedroom door so she would not be awakened from her nap when the others came in from their lunch time. That was about 12:30 P.M. I usually let her sleep for several hours and when I went into the bedroom to wake her up from her nap, she was laying on the floor. I forgot to pull her barrier up. She was awake and I struggled to pick her up from the floor. Little by little I got her up and pulled her to my chest with my arms under her arms and we fell back on the hospital bed. I gradually moved her to one side of the bed and rolled her off of me. I had to change her dirty diapers and get her cleaned up and put her on the Jerry chair. Then I brought her into the living room to watch television. I should have put the rails up, but she hardly ever moves, so I did not think she would roll over and fall to the floor. She looked so pitiful looking up at me from the floor. I don't know how long she had been laying there. God was gracious and Nell did not break anything as far as I can tell so far. I feel so alone when something like this happens. The children are so busy that I don't want to call them.

11/23/2017   Thursday, Thanksgiving Day. I gave Shantel the day off, so I cleaned Nell and got her dressed this morning. After she fell off the bed yesterday, as I was moving her around this morning it appeared to me that she was unsure about her safety. It is a beautiful Thanksgiving Day. We are all going to have Thanksgiving Dinner today at Carrie's house. That is Billy, Kim and Carrie and several of their children who are not committed to their in-laws for Thanksgiving will be there. Nell and I spent the afternoon at Carrie's house for thanksgiving. When I got ready to leave, Laurel came up to Nell as I was wheeling her out in the wheel chair. Laurel said, "I love you." And Nannie responded with "I love you" with her lips, but no words. Calvin and I had a hard time getting Nell into my car and getting her out of the car and on the Jerry Chair at our home.

11/24/2017   Saturday. I got Nell up this morning, cleaned her, and dressed her then brought her out to the living room where she could be among her children who came for breakfast. Kim and Pat stayed overnight and Carrie and Calvin came for breakfast. Nell had wet the bed so bad through her Depends I had to strip the bed and wash the sheets. After her nap today, I fed her a glass of milkshake. She lifted her left hand as if to hold the glass, so I let her. She took hold of the glass and tried to lift it to her lips. When she got near her mouth she puckered up her lips to drink. At this point I had to help lift up the glass to her lips so she could drink. I was surprised! She hadn't been able to move her arms to any degree for six months. But she wanted to hold the glass and drink the drink by herself. Nell and I watched the Iron Bowl today

She did not show any emotion or interest in the game. At times her head would turn to the side and she would just stare at some object or nothing but stare she would with seemingly little awareness. When I would talk with her right into her eyes she would show some animation. Her eyes would widen and eyebrows would go up.

I watched the Alabama vs Auburn game today, pretty much by myself. I made some hamburgers, potatoes and salad thinking that I would have company who said they would come and watch the game with me. I got to thinking about that. I have a lot of friends, relatives, and Christian brothers from church who Nell and I used to watch the ballgames with, but now with just me, it is too much trouble, near impossible, for me to take Nell anywhere. I need to stay with her, and so I will watch the games by myself.

11/27/2017   I asked Jan, Kindred Hospice Nurse, if I could try a Hoya lift to help me get Nell from the Jerry chair to her portable potty and from the potty to bed. I have been sensing a slight pain in my lower back. They delivered it but not with the fabric with a potty hole in it. They are to deliver that today.

11/28/2017   Toni came and bathed & dressed Nell this morning.

11/29/2017   I tried to put Nell to bed last night using the Hoya Lift. It had the potty hole in it. The whole process was too difficult. I may return it today.

11/30/2017   Thursday. I haven't made any notes the last few days. I ordered a Hoya Lift through Kindred Care Hospice. I tried to lift Nell from the Jerry chair to the portable potty, and then to bed. It was not an easy task. I told Jan the nurse from Kindred Care Hospice, the next day and she told me that the lift was made to put her in bed and from the bed to the chair. But the fabric had a hole in it for use of the potty, but it was too hard to use. I told Jan and asked her to have it returned, but she said to keep it and it may come in good use later. Yesterday, Nell seemed to be more lifeless, although at times her eyes were open and bright. She did eat her Ensure but not with much expressed appetite.

It takes about 45 minutes to get Nell in bed and ready for sleep. She starts out on the portable potty. I move the Jerry chair in position and remove her lower clothes, then I pick her up and turn 180 degrees and sit her on the portable potty. I leave her there for about 15 minutes to see if she can have a bowel movement. Meanwhile, I take off the upper clothes and put on her night gown. She usually has a bowel movement, so I clean her and put her in bed. I put the hospital bed on the lowest position in order to move her from the potty to the bed by turning her 90 degrees and setting her on the bed, then I lay her in position. I jack the hospital bed to the highest so I don't have to lean over and I get her ready to sleep. I clean her more thoroughly and put some barrier salve on her bottom. She has a hemorroid and that has to be treated with Preparation H. Then I put on her Depends. I pull the covers up on her, then the side rail. I put eye drops in her eyes because they have had an infection. Then I hook up the oxygen hose to her nose. She is now ready for sleep.

I have tried to keep the bedroom and the whole house from having a nursing home smell, but my daughter Kim, said that there was a slight smell from Nell's nightgowns when I put them in the dirty clothes hamper. She suggested I fill the washing machine with some water and soap and drop the used gowns into the washing machine rather than in the dirty clothes hamper. That would eliminate the possibility of the urine smell from the night clothes in the hamper.

Nell has been a little lifeless the last few days. I detect it in her eyes, mostly. Her appetite has diminished somewhat lately. She is drinking all the Ensure when I give it to her, but she is less interested in drinking it. I have to keep touching her lips with the straw, and telling her to sip on the straw. It helps a little. It takes longer to feed her than in the past.

Nell was reared in a loving home as the only child. Her older sister went to Alabama University when Nell was a teenager. All the relatives spoiled her. She has no relatives who are close to her to help take care of her. She has children and grand-children, and they are busy with their own lives. I think about her parents who would want their daughter well taken care of at a time like this with her disease of Alzheimer's. I hope they know, somehow, that the man who married their daughter is taking care of her. She is helpless. Maybe they are cheering me on from their place in heaven. I need cheering on.

12/5/2017   Tuesday. It has been a few days since I have entered any events in my diary of Nell's Caregiving husband. She was visited by the Kindred Care Hospice nurse on Monday. She took Nell's vitals and all was well. Sunday night during the night between the hours of 1:30 A.M. Monday A.M. and 6:00 A.M. Nell pushed the oxygen from her nose up over her eyes. I think that could be hurtful and damaging. The protrusions that go into her nose that feeds her the oxygen are hard pieces and could damage her eyes. I don't know how she did it when she can barely move her arms. During these last few days, you can tell that her life force has deteriorated. She has had difficulty sucking on a straw, so I tip a glass up for her to drink. She wants to sleep. Then at times she stays awake while she watches TV, and during the program she might turn her head and just stare. During the night when I check to see if the oxygen is hooked up properly and she has enough covers, and when she wakes and looks at me there is a fear in her eyes as if she is looking at a stranger. When I wake her up in the morning she looks like she is looking at a stranger. During the day when I talk to her she looks like she is looking at a stranger. When I clean her from a bowel movement and put her in bed, she looks like she is looking at a stranger.

12/6/2017   Wed. Last night Nell moved off her pillow and was laying on her side. Unusual, because she usually does not move at all when she lays down.

12/7/2017   Last night Nell turned on her right side facing the wall. Her face was hidden between the mattress and the wall. About 1:30 AM I moved her back on her pillow. At 4:00 AM when I got up she had laid back in that same position against the wall. She was also damp with sweat, and had scrubbed the back of her hand on the wall and blood was running down the wall.

12/9/2017   Saturday. Nell had a troublesome night last night. I try to put pillows against the pull-up barrier and one against the wall so she will not scrub herself. But the night before last, she scrubbed her hand on the wall even around the pillow and she bled against the wall quite an amount. Last night she kept kicking her left leg as she layed on her back and got her leg caught in the rails on the pull-up barrier. I woke up about 1:00 A.M. and noticed this and got her leg untangled and placed another pillow against the rail. At 4:00 A.M. she had it against the rail again. When I woke her up this morning about 7:00 A.M. to wash her and dress her, I noticed her left leg was all red and on the side of her leg there was bleeding in a couple of places where she had scraped it against the pull-up barrier. (From this moment on, I put pillows against the wall and against the barrier, and duct taped the pillows so she could not move the pillows and injure her legs.) Concerning her eating Ensure at her meal times and drinking her orange juice in the morning, it is getting harder to put the straw in her mouth when she purses her lips to refuse it. Or if I try to get her to drink out of a glass, she will purse her lips to let me know that she doesn't want to drink. She actually does this in an angry manner. Like she is telling me, "I don't want to drink. Quit forcing that glass in my lips." I take it away and wait a few minutes and try again. I may have to do that several times, until I get her to drink all her juice or the Ensure. It may take 15 to 30 minutes.

Nell just wanted to sleep today and she did not have any energy. She was quite lifeless and layed over in her Jerry chair. When I put her on the couch after lunch for her nap, she fell off the couch on to the floor. She curled up on the floor and when I looked at the couch she didn't appear in sight and I thought she walked off somewhere, knowing that she could not walk, so when I got closer to the couch, I saw her on the floor. It was difficult for me to pick her up to put her on the couch, then from the couch to the Jerry chair. She was pitiful. She had no expression about the whole incident. I sat beside her on the couch and spoke to her for a few minutes, not knowing if any of the conversation got through to her. I told her that I was finding it hard to take care of her and keeping her safe. I said, "I wanted to care for you as long as I could. If it becomes beyond my ability I will have to take you to a nursing home. I know you don't want to go to a nursing home." I don't think any of that registered with her. She could not comprehend what I was saying.

After I put her in the Jerry chair, she threw her legs to one side where I had a pillow to protect her from any further injury on the leg that was already in bad shape. I have to watch her where ever I put her, because she will find ways to fall out on the floor. Or get scrubbed on the barrier rail on the bed. I put a pillow to guard her leg tonight and taped the pillow to the rail so she could not kick it off. I put a pillow against the wall so she will not scrub herself on the wall.

12/10/2017 Sunday. Nell slept very deep and did not move as I could tell. The pillow taped to the barrier seemed to work. I had a hard time feeding her this morning. She is not drinking through the straw very well. She will not suck more than a couple of swallows and then she lets the liquid go down her throat, and will not suck any more. I have to put the Ensure in a glass and let her sip it. When I put the Ensure against her lips she will sip and drink. That is the way I had to do it last night and this morning. Another thing I noticed lately is that she brings her knees up and wants to lay on her side. She does not want to straighten out her legs and lay on her back as she has in the past. She does not want to fold her legs and lay on her back, unless I put a pillow to help hold her legs up.

12/12/2017 Tuesday. The last several days have been scary. Nell will not drink her Ensue with a straw. She will just sip it from a glass, and is very slow. One time she had a mouthful and before she swallowed it, she coughed and spit the mouthful out. Today, she drank a total of 2 cans of Ensure out of a small glass for the day. It took a long time to feed her. Normally she drinks three glasses of Ensure a day. She lays her head to the left side, in bed and also, when she is in the Jerry Chair. I put her in bed early tonight. She was in bed around 5:30 P.M. Normally she has a bowel movement, but nothing tonight. She was very shaky to sit on the portable potty alone tonight. She leaned to one side and closed her eyes. I was afraid she would fall off the potty chair. I don't know how much longer I can sit her on the potty chair. It was difficult getting her out of her chair onto the potty, and then from the potty onto the bed. She went to sleep quite soon when I put her to bed. Her eyes were so droopy and the whites of her eyes were a slight brownish rather than the white that contrasts with her blue eyes. I put some eye drops in her eyes. Tomorrow is Wednesday and I usually go to Senior Choir Rehearsal. I don't know if I will go to choir tomorrow, Nell looks so bad. It worries me to leave. Andrea is coming to stay with her tomorrow, and if I stay, she can help me care for Nell and will be helpful as I try to minister to Nell. I just don't want to be alone with Nell tomorrow, so even if I stay, I think I will let Andrea come to stay also. Nell looks too bad. If she is looking better in the morning, I may feel I can go to choir rehearsal.

12/13/2017   Nell seemed better this morning, and so I will go to choir rehearsal. When I returned she was her normal self. Andrea said she did well during the day. Nell is not sucking her Ensure through a straw. Yesterday she sipped her juice and Ensure very slowly, sometimes refusing. It took some time to feed her at the meal times. One time she had a mouthful and coughed it out. She lays with her head at the left side.

12/14/2017   Thursday. Nell slept very soundly last night. She drank her orange juice very slowly; she finally drank her Ensure. She would not drink it with a straw, but sipped it slowly. Andrea stayed with Nell while I played golf in a Minister's tournament at Timber Creek. When I returned home about 4:30 P.M. I started feeding her the evening Ensure. She drank it all with a straw, and she drank it like she was hungry. I put her on the portable potty tonight. She was compacted and I had to help her have a bowel movement. I cleaned her up and dressed the sore on her tail bone where she tore some skin last night when she sat on the potty. When I was carrying her to the potty, she usually helps with some weight on her legs, but, she just dropped and her tail bone hit the potty hard. When I began to clean her to put on her Depends, I noticed the blood. I treated the wound and put a band aid on it. I had a very hard time picking her up from the Jerry chair to the portable potty, and putting her from the potty to the bed tonight. She does not help at all. I have to carry her from under her arms to the potty, and then from the potty to the bed. I may have to start using the lift to put her in bed from the Jerry chair, and not use the potty. Jan, the nurse, told me yesterday that Nell was slipping badly. She was telling me that I need to be aware that she is going to die soon. She has been staring a lot the last several days. Yesterday, I showed her a Christmas card that Luana sent to us. She looked at it and when I moved it from one side to the other, she followed the movement of the card. She looked as if she was trying to get closer to the card to read the writings. When I checked to see if all was well with her about 1:30 AM this morning she opened her eyes. This morning when I checked her oxygen she did not wake up, she was sound asleep.

12/15/2017   Friday. Nell slept well all night. Did not toss and turn like several nights ago. During the day she lays her head to the left and just stares. Did not eat any juice or Ensure. Andrea could not get her to eat.

12/16/2017   Saturday. Yesterday was the entering of a new stage in the caregiving of Nell's Alzheimer's disease. She is refusing to drink the Ensure. She would sip a mouthful then she would cough and spit it up. She is getting weak. I tried to put her on the potty last night and I was not able to carry her full weight, so I layed her on the bed. From now on there will be no more portable potty. I cannot carry her in a 180 degree turn from the Jerry chair to the potty. I can make a 90 degree turn to the bed. That is what I did. So I put her in bed and cleaned her and treated a sore she got from my last attempt to put her on the potty, and she sat hard on the potty and broke open the skin near her tail bone. This morning I did not try to get her out of bed. I am unable to put her in the Jerry chair and dress her, so I just cleaned her, put on her Depends, took off her wet night clothes and put on a new gown to lay her in bed. So, she is just confined to bed, unless I am able to use the Hoya lift. But she seems too weak for me to try to use the Hoya lift. I tried to use the Hoya lift several days ago, and it was too difficult for me and for her. Now today (Saturday) Her eyes are weak. She drank a very small amount of orange juice with Miralax in it. It took some time. But she did not drink any Ensure. It is now 11:00 A.M. and almost time for her noon Ensure and she has not drank her morning Ensure. I am concerned that it won't be long before God calls her home. At the most a week at this pace of her eating and not getting any liquids in her.

Carrie came by last night (Friday) to talk to me about the funeral arrangements. What I wanted and what the children wanted. So we will work it out. It is now near 5:00 P.M., and Nell still has not eaten any Ensure today, only some of the orange juice this morning with Miralax. I called Jan, the Kindred Hospice Nurse. No answer, left a text message of the situation. She called back several times, but I was charging the phone and did not hear her call. I called back and she did not answer.

12/17/2017   Sunday. God called Nell to come be with Him in her heavenly home about 6:30 P.M.

12/18/2017   Monday (1:30 AM) Nell left this earth and presence of early loved ones last night at 6:30 P.M. after several days of not eating any Ensure or orange juice or water. Friday morning she had about a half of a glass of orange Juice. She would not drink any Ensure Friday, Saturday and Sunday morning and noon and during the evening she died. The last several days, when myself or Andrea, her caregiver, attempted to feed her Ensue, she would take a mouthful and cough it up. Or she would purse her lips and not take any Ensure. I made milkshakes of different flavors hoping that she would taste the milkshake and then drink a glass of milkshake, but she wouldn't. The nurse had warned me not to force a drink on her or she might aspirate.

Carrie came over Sunday afternoon and said she was going to stay the night with me, because Nell looked so bad. She called Billy and he said he was going to come over and stay the evening with me. Carrie's children, and grandchildren came to sing Christmas carols to Nannie. They all came over to eat a chicken dinner and sing. I had been sitting beside Nell Saturday, and Sunday when I came home from Church and held her hand so she did not feel alone, if she had that kind of thoughts. I don't know, but I did not want to leave the room but to make sure she sensed my presence or was in her view, anyway. So, Sunday afternoon about 6:00 P.M. we were all in the bedroom around Nell's bed. I was holding her hand beside her bed. Carrie had left the room for a few minutes and about 6:30 P.M. she came back into the room and made a remark to me that Nell looked very white. A few moments before, Nell had made a slight cough, and that, I think, is when she took her last breath and her heart had stopped. When Carrie noticed her white complexion, I tried to feel her pulse, but I couldn't feel it except a couple of beats, then nothing. A couple of beats, then nothing. I determined then, that she had expired. The Lord had come and took her soul to be with Him until that great Resurrection Day. Carrie had called Billy earlier and had suggested he come over to be with Nell with the rest of the local family. Billy arrived about 15 minutes after Nell had breathed her last, and embraced her emotionally.

I phoned the Kindred Care Hospice and they sent a nurse to pronounce her death. She called Mobile Memorial Gardens, and they sent an ambulance to come get her body and take it to the funeral home. Her physical presence in this home is no more. Her physical presence to me and to our family will no longer be the joy of years gone by. She has gone into the presence of those who belong to God through Jesus Christ, and to the saints who have gone on before her. She has joined her mother, father and her sister in the heavenlies.

12/19/2017   Tuesday. Yesterday, Bill, Carrie and I went to Mobile Memorial Gardens to make the funeral arrangements for Nell. We had a prepaid funeral policy, so it was a minimal cost to make the plans, both in the funeral home and at the cemetery. The funeral plans are set for Thursday (12/21) at 12:00 P.M. at Dauphin Way Baptist Church. Interment at Mobile Memorial Gardens afterwards, then a fellowship meal for family and close friends at our house at 28 Chase Cir. in Saraland. It is lonely without Nell's presence in the home. Yesterday Bill suggested we go have breakfast at Waffle house. The first thought was: "I can't leave Nell. I have to find a caregiver to take care of Nell while I leave." I am psychologically tied to her care. It felt so different to get my senses and realize I was unchained from this voluntary bondage of caregiving. As I look back, there were so many times I was going to put Nell in a nursing home. It was too hard. I had put up some caregiving problems that when they came, I could not do, that would force me to put her in a nursing home. But God was gracious and gave me the ability, health and strength to meet the need when it came, and I continued to care for her through all the difficulties. Thank God, He took her when He did, because she had quit eating and it was difficult to see her waste away in a terrible weak condition. She would just look at me with her forlorn eyes. There was nothing I could do. I sat beside her, holding her hand, the children and grandchildren were getting ready to sing Christmas Carols to her when she coughed a small quiet cough. I didn't know she had died, until Carrie noticed her color. I took her pulse and there was several beats, then nothing, several beats, then nothing. By then, we could all see that God came and took her, the hour of His choosing. "Thank You God! You were merciful to her, and to us."

Billy, Carrie and I went to Mobile Memorial Gardens on Monday and made all the arrangements for the funeral to be held at Dauphin Way Baptist Church on Thursday, Dec. 21, at 12:00 P.M, visitation from 10 to 12, and family visitation from 9:30 A.M. to 10:00 A.M. We had decided that if they did a good job in preparing Nell to look like Nell from a picture we gave them, we would have an open casket during visitation. However, after we viewed Nell in the casket, we decided to close the casket for public visitation. The service lasted about an hour and 15 minutes. We all made comment on the service and the auditorium was beautifully decorated for Christmas. After the interment, guests and family came to my house for a fellowship meal provided by the church family.

12/23/2017   Saturday. It is one day short of a week since Nell went to be with God in Paradise. This week has been a hazy remembrance for me. I was going to wait until after Christmas to make some notes in the diary, but decided to make these notes today, thinking, I may not remember what I want to say, next week, after Christmas. A number of people have called me. I have been thankful for their caring. I was hurting terribly after a year of 24 hour care to Nell who did not relate, nor respond. It has been a year since she has uttered more than a few words, and six months no words at all. When I would look into her eyes to speak to her, there was not any response. She would turn her head and stare at something. I would talk to her anyway. I would pray with her at night when I got her into bed. There didn't seem to be any response. But now that she is gone, I miss her presence even though there was no relating. She was pitiful, and was my master. She was helpless. I was bound to her day and night. I wanted to be her caregiver till God came and rescued her from this darkness of mind, and helpless body. All I can remember now is not the 63 years of marriage, but the last several years of caregiving and watching her go down, watching her deteriorate in mind and body until she would not eat. It was two and a half days with no food and water, when her heart stopped beating. She was in darkness, and at that moment I like to think she came into the light of awareness again. I like to think that her mother and dad and her sister welcomed her and said, "Well, Bill did take care of you until you escaped that torment and joined us." I pray that God said to me, "Well done my good and faithful servant." I pray that I will hear Him and can be lifted out of my grief and tears, which are on the edge of my emotions.

One thing that has irritated me is the way well meaning people try to minister to me during my hurt is not listen to me. They want to tell me about their relatives who had this disease. They want to give me all their advice that God is with me, and Nell is in a better place. But they don't want to listen to me. I just quit trying to talk and explain my hurt, and listen to them. I wish I could sort out my feelings. I will have to do it without any help from others. When they leave or hang up I am alone again. God, be with me.

12/24/2017   Sunday. I came to Bill's home on Saturday. Two days after funeral. We will be going to Jackson to be with Will and Bethany. We will attend worship with Will at his church today and return to Bill's home afterward. We attended worship at the church where Will and Bethany worship. Will played the drums during the worship time and did such a fine job. Came back to Big Level and went to bed Christmas Eve. Had a restless night's rest. May be the new norm. What to do?

To Nell:

> I think about what you are doing today? Worship with Jesus? Fellowship with Family? Being your joyful self in Paradise? We remember you today. Don't forget me. Rode to Jackson, Ms. with Bill, Nita and Mick. We went to Will & Bethany's Church. Had Sunday dinner with Will & Bethany at their lovely home. Will showed Bill, Mick and I the place and equipment of the Country Club where he works. Had a good day with family. It was a long drive. Made it alright. I have a habit of looking for you in

situations where using manners to let you go first is my response. You left me last week at about this time of the evening on Sunday. I thank God you were called. It was pitiful the way you were wasting away. I want to cry. I was helpless to you. It was best you left to be with God and the saints who went on before. I think sometimes, from where you are if you would let yourself be known to me to give me some assurance that I did right for you in my care-giving. I feel like crying now. I have to write this down to explain my feelings. I hurt and am lonely even though you did not respond, you were present. People call and give me a lot of spiritual advice, and tell me about their loved one's who died from Alzheimer's but won't let me explain the feelings of my heart. They are kind to phone, and their motives are pure. You were a wonderful wife. I will express my feelings tomorrow.

12/25/2017   Monday, Christmas Day.

I am at Billy's home in Big Level. I am still in bed. It is about 5:00 AM. I am on the edge of crying on this day, remembering how this day was so special to you. You put a lot into it, buying gifts for the next Christmas on Dec. 26. You were so careful to make sure everyone was petted. Even the Christmas meal was planned so meticulously and ahead of time, and especially the stuffed mushrooms. How you protected them when they came out of the oven. But when you weren't looking I sneaked one, or two. I remember how nonchalant you tried to be sitting back watching the children opening their presents. You could not open yours because you were going from one child to the other seeing the surprise and joy on each face. You went to bed late to make sure all was in place for Santa's arrival, and was up before the children so you could greet them at the tree with a mountain of gifts to hand out. But, at the appropriate time. We will miss you today as we celebrate Christmas. But we really missed you last year also, but at least you were present. Can you see today? At every family member's home today your presence will be missed. I am crying again. I am worried as I watch Billy and Nita and Mick open their presents that I will be too emotional in that you are not here. I am going to get out of bed, take a shower and join them in the living room. Maybe that will sober me up to meet them and celebrate Christ's birthday, all because of you.

I came home from Billy's and went to share Christmas with Carrie's family and Billy. Had a great Christmas Dinner and opening of presents with Carrie's family. I don't want to get in an unhealthy state of mind, but it's Christmas, maybe I'll allow myself some nostalgia. Can I pretend you have gone on a trip and I am writing to tell you what happened today? Carrie and Calvin's family opened presents like when our family all gathered to open presents. You set the tradition. You should have seen the joy on the children, especially the grandchildren and great grandchildren. You would have been proud of Carrie's Christmas dinner. I think I am going to cry. I should have gone on the trip and you stayed to enjoy this season with the children. You were so much more loving, interested and helpful at Christmas than me. You were cheated, and I got all the blessings. Makes me feel guilty because you deserve all the blessings of Christmas, and not me. You were the one who brought Christ into our family and then you leave. The very one who started it all, and I get the blessings.

I mentioned earlier that I told Nell's parents when we left their home in 1954, that I would take care of her. Her parents were crying. They had one daughter who lived up in Long Island, New York and now I am taking their little girl. It broke their hearts. I told them I would take care of her. Off we drove in our little Chevrolet coupe to Cherry Point, N. C. our first duty station as a Marine Pilot. She was so young and inexperienced as a housewife. Several months ago she wrote about her dating, marriage and life with me before she went into the darkness. She told about her love for me. I was ashamed that I did not show more affection, love, and regular gift giving. But several weeks ago, I looked into her eyes and told her, "I told your mom and dad when we married that I would take care of you and I have, haven't I? She showed no response. I made a covenant with God, that I would do my best every day. I prayed that covenant prayer to God every day. I could not take any shortcuts to her care after I made that prayer, because I would feel like a hypocrite.

2018

1/6/2018   I have tried to edit my daily journey with Nell these last few days, notes that were written, during this last 18 months. It has been difficult to go through it again. When I read of those experiences, I got sick to my stomach. I have hesitated to get back to it again. I have looked at pictures of Nell in the progress of this disease. It tears me apart to see my sweet lovely wife to daily get more helpless, and her appearance causes tears to my eyes.

1/8/2018   Monday 1:58 A.M. I am going through a difficult time trying to get on in life. Yesterday at church, I felt a lot of comfort on the part of the people in S.S. and in worship. But when you are hurting you feel that you need more comforting than what you are getting. I feel a lot of the members want you to begin doing ministries that you may not be ready to do. There is a need and they feel I can fill that need, but I don't feel I have grieved to where I feel comfortable in leading in certain areas. If I am upfront in leading and try to be encouraging and upbeat, I feel like I am pretending, because I do not feel upbeat. But I don't want to be up front leading a SS dept in a state of grief. I really don't feel upbeat. I felt so bad yesterday afternoon, suicide even entered my mind. Decision making for my life which is nearly over after 87 years, even though God has given me good health, I didn't feel there was much ahead of me, in life. Family have their interests. Friends have their interest. Your companion in life has gone on ahead, so why continue here?

1/9/2018   Tuesday. Several ministers invited me to lunch on Thursday and a game of golf at Timber Creek (Art Burroughs, Charles Gibbs, JamesMercer). I find that concern for me to be helpful in my grief. A grief person at Kindred Hospice, Cathy Wyatt will meet with me on Wednesday. 1/11/2018. Cathy was a good counselor. She was very helpful.

1/17/2018   I went to the cemetery. They did not have the headstone in place as yet. The attendant said it was too cold and there were so many funerals. I told him not to worry about it, Nell was not there. She was in the heavenlies.

2/17/2018   I went to the cemetery to commemorate Nell's being gone from this earthly presence two months to be with Jesus Christ. I put flowers in the container on the headstone. It is still hard to not weep at times. I sense Nell's presence. I had a dream two nights ago, where I held Nell's hand with my right hand and we were walking down the sidewalk of a shopping mall. She was wearing a flowered dress of many colors. She was radiant, and full of joy with her blonde hair flowing in the breeze. It only lasted some seconds, it seemed.

5/6/2018   Sunday, I slipped backwards going into the shower and tried to stop my fall with the left elbow and broke my arm just under the left joint ball. When I tried to get up my arm just dangled in pain. I could only get relief by laying on my back. When I fell, I hit the bathroom door and closed it, so I couldn't get out. It took about an hour to figure how to open the door without much pain. I got the door open and slithered out like a worm and pulled my Ipad off the nightstand and sent a text message to my daughter down the street to come help me and call 911. I fell at 6:00 A.M. and finally got to emergency at 7:30 A.M .

During the first four weeks of recovery, my daughter and son-in-law helped me shower and dress and eat. My daughter stayed with me at night. I was able to take care of myself in four weeks, but the next few weeks were difficult trying to take care of my needs. It is July 16, 2018 and I am about 90 % healed. I had carpal tunnel surgery on my right hand during my healing. My left hand is numb and tingling on the fingers, and so is my right hand, which makes it hard for me to function.

7/15/2018   Sunday, Carrie's family and I went to dinner after church and then to the cemetery and sang Happy Birthday to Nell at the gravesite to observe Nell's first birthday in heaven.

ABOUT THE AUTHOR

Born in North Dakota in 1930, Bill Whitfield's family moved to Visalia, California in 1930. He graduated from Visalia Union High School in 1948 and received an Associate of Arts degree from Oceanside-Carlsbad Junior College in 1951. He joined the military during the Korean War where he served in Guam and Okinawa, then entered the Naval Aviation Cadet program at Pensacola, and was commissioned a Second Lt., in the U. S. Marine Corps in October, 1954. Bill married Miss Nelda Pugh on October 23, 1954, a graduate of Murphy High School, class of 1953 at Dauphin Way Baptist Church, in Mobile, Ala.

During his time of training in the U.S Navy, Cadet Whitfield flew a number of planes, such as the SNJ, T-28, F4F, TV-2, F9F Panther jet, and in Marine Squadron VMF 334, the FJ-2 Fury, and also the flying boxcar, the R4Q, while assigned to MAG 32. After he was released from active duty he was a sales and flight instructor of Cessna aircraft at Fullerton, California. He was saved and Baptized at the First Southern Baptist Church in Fullerton, California in 1959. Bill worked as a salesman at United Desk Co in Los Angeles , California. He surrendered to the Gospel Ministry in 1965 and returned with his family to Mobile, Alabama, and received his Bachelor of Arts degree at Mobile College in 1968. He continued his education by attending The Southern Baptist Theological Seminary in Louisville, Kentucky where he received the Masters of Theology degree, in 1971. He then earned the Doctor of Ministry degree at The New Orleans Southern Baptist Theological Seminary in New Orleans, Louisiana, in 1978, while pastoring Cypress Shores Baptist Church in Mobile, Al. where he was called in 1971.

Dr. Whitfield was the organizing pastor at Cypress Shores Baptist Church, until December 1992. He pastored several churches as interim pastor, and went on staff part time at Dauphin Way Baptist Church from June 1998, until August, 2016, when he resigned to become the full time caregiver to his wife of 63 years, when she was released into the merciful hands of God, from the terrible Alzheimer's disease. He and Nell parented three children, nine grandchildren and fourteen great grandchildren.

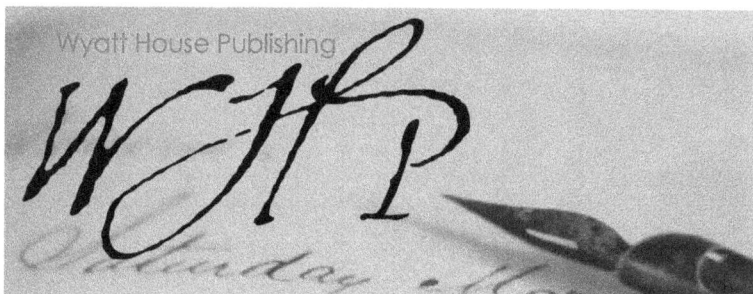

www.ingramcontent.com/pod-product-compliance
Lightning Source LLC
LaVergne TN
LVHW091217080426
835509LV00009B/1034